Lemons

HUNDREDS OF
HOUSEHOLD HINTS

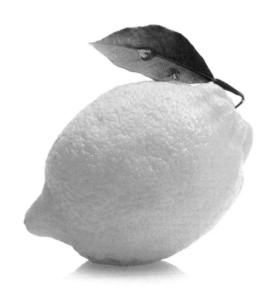

Publisher's Note:
All reasonable care has been exercised by the author and publisher to ensure that the tips and remedies included in this guide are simple and safe. However, it is important to note that all uses of lemons should be practised with caution and a doctor's, or relevant professional's, advice should be sought if in any doubt or before any topical or medicinal usage – the advice in this book is not a replacement for that of a doctor. The author, editors and publisher take no responsibility for any consequences of any application which results from reading the information contained herein.

A note on measurements:
Please note also that the measurements provided in this book are presented as metric/imperial/US-cups practical equivalents, and that all eggs are medium (UK)/large (US) respectively unless otherwise stated.

This is a **FLAME TREE** book
First published in 2011

Publisher and Creative Director: Nick Wells
Senior Project Editor: Catherine Taylor
Picture Research: Charlotte McLean and Catherine Taylor
Art Director: Mike Spender
Layout Design: Jane Ashley
Digital Design and Production: Chris Herbert
Proofreader: Alison Hill
Indexer: Helen Snaith

Special thanks to Laura Bulbeck.

13 15 14 12

3 5 7 9 10 8 6 4 2

This edition first published in 2011 by
FLAME TREE PUBLISHING
Crabtree Hall, Crabtree Lane
Fulham, London SW6 6TY
United Kingdom

www.flametreepublishing.com

Flame Tree is part of The Foundry Creative Media Co. Ltd
© 2011 this edition The Foundry Creative Media Co. Ltd

ISBN 978-0-85775-262-8

A CIP Record for this book is available from the British Library upon request.

Printed in China

The images on pages 151–81 are © Foundry Arts. All other images are courtesy of Shutterstock.com and © the following contributors: 1 & 102 Viktar Malyshchyts; 3 & 10 & 109t maragu; 5l & 19b & 128 Robin W; 5r & 131t, 115 Yuri Arcurs; 6 ODM; 7 Igor Dutina; 8 Magdalena Bujak; 9 Colour; 11 Olaf Speier; 13 Tischenko Irina; 14 Ziga Cetrtic; 15, 41, 106, 130t matka_Wariatka; 17 maria17; 18 Elena Ray; 19t Konstantin Sutyagin; 21 Itinerant Lens; 22t Senol Yaman; 22b Tamara Kulikova; 23r Natalia D.; 23l tan4ikk; 24 fredredhat; 25 Taratorki; 26 Cheryl E. Davis; 26 mates; 27t Alistair Cotton; 27b Evgeny Tomeev; 28 Dmitry Naumov; 29 Sandra Cunningham; 31 Elena Elisseeva; 32 Yurchyks; 33b Joe Gough; 33t ronstik; 34 Sam72; 35 VVO; 36 Katerina Havelkova; 37 Grauvision; 39 Ambient Ideas; 40b SeDmi; 40t trailexplorers; 42 zirconicusso; 43b cosma; 43t Joe Cox; 45b John Kasawa; 45t Vasily Topko; 46 ID1974; 47 terekhov igor; 49, 140t Mike Flippo; 50 Cattallina; 51 Ivaschenko Roman; 52t ostill; 53 Blend Images; 54 Africa Studios; 55t David W. Leindecker; 55b Vladimir Melnik; 56 & 192 Graeme Dawes; 57 Joy Brown; 59 Svetlana Larina; 60 ER_09; 61l Adisa; 61r Jackiso; 62 Balazs Justin; 63 imagestalk; 64 Martin Novak; 65b, 104 marilyn barbone; 65t Wiktory; 67 Nessi; 68b Fong Kam Yee; 68t Subbotina Anna; 69 Dave Allen Photography; 70 Jorg Hackemann; 71t Liliya Kulianionak; 71b psnoonan; 73 Lusoimages; 74 guigaamartins; 75 Annette Shaff; 76 Sashkin; 77 Studio Barcelona; 79, 83, 87 Valua Vitaly; 80 Artpose Adam Borkowski; 81 PixAchi; 82l kzww; 82r sergojpg; 84 Ariusz Nawrocki; 85l nastiakru; 85r Penny Hillcrest; 86 Quayside; 88 Phil Date; 89 Lana K; 90 Yuganov Konstantin; 91 vgstudio; 92 Irina1977; 93 Ivanova Inga; 94t Rick P Lewis; 94b Tania Zbrodko; 95 Margaret M Stewart; 97 Elena Kharichkina; 98r dionisvera; 98l Kalim; 99 Goodluz; 100 Vadim Ponomarenko; 101b aspen rock; 101t Leah-Anne Thompson; 103 lenetstan; 105 Stuart Miles; 107t AISPIX; 107b Vinicius Tupinamba; 108 NatalieJean; 109b Ronald Sumners; 110 librakv; 111, 135, 147 Lilyana Vynogradova; 112, 144 Christopher Elwell; 113 sixninepixels; 114 Juri Arcurs; 116 artur gabrysiak; 117 Gorilla; 118t newphotoservice; 118b Selecstock; 119 Blaj Gabriel; 120 Christian Delbert; 121 wavebreakmedia ltd; 122 design56; 123 Volosina; 124t Andrei Mihalcea; 124b Piotr Marcinski; 125 Volodymyr Burdiak; 126t BeaB; 126b Faiz Zaki; 127l Brooke Becker; 127r kiboka; 129 Aleksandar Todorovic; 130b kostudio; 131b Sandi; 132 Donald R. Swartz; 133 inacio pires; 136t Paul Reid; 137 area381; 138t Olga Utlyakova; 139t Elzbieta Sekowska; 140b tacar; 141 Paul Cowan; 142t Marie C Fields; 142b Peter zijlstra; 143t B.G. Smith; 143b Gemenacom; 145 buriy; 146 Elke Dennis; 148 Monkey Business Images; 149 trgowanlock; 182 Hallgerd; 183 iofoto; 185t James Steidl; 185b Victor Newman; 186 stavklem; 187 Dino O.; 188 Jiri Hera; 189 jurasy.

Lemons

HUNDREDS OF
HOUSEHOLD HINTS

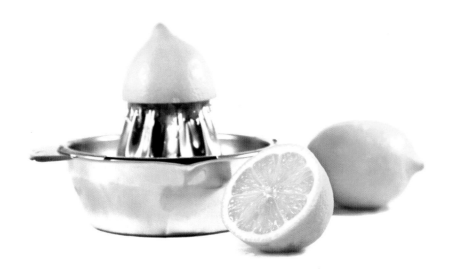

Diane & Jon Sutherland

**FLAME TREE
PUBLISHING**

Contents

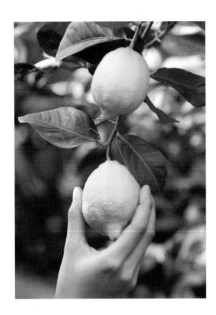
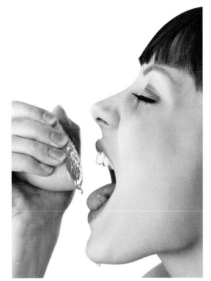

Introduction

The bright yellow lemon, with its unmistakable citrus smell, is hugely versatile. Its value as a preservative and for flavouring has long been recognized, but it also has enormous potential in the home; as a beauty product, for health benefits and as a natural cleaning product. It is possible to use every part of the lemon; the juice is rich in fruit acids and natural sugars and for generations it has been used as a remedy for chills and coughs, as well as to ease sunburn and skin rashes.

The Lemon Tree

The *Citrus Limon*, or the lemon tree, is an evergreen that was originally native to Asia, and particularly to India, Burma and China. The tree is now grown throughout Europe and many

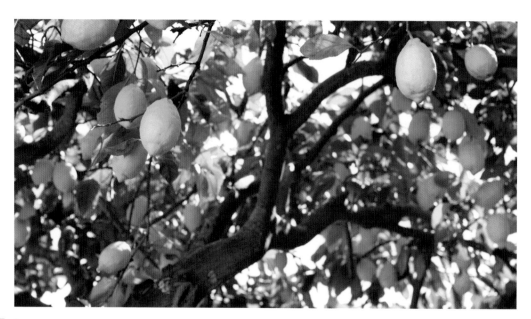

other sub-tropical climates, including Arizona and California in the United States. Its oval, fresh-smelling, yellow fruit is popular around the world. It has the added advantage that it bears fruit all year round, and selective cultivation has created dozens of different varieties.

The lemon tree needs warmth and sunshine, good drainage and regular watering. Cultivated trees are regularly pruned and bees are encouraged, as they are essential to pollinate the flowers.

The Versatile Lemon

Although lemons are used commercially for the production of soft drinks and food flavourings, their use in the home has often been limited to culinary use and for adding to drinks. But tangy lemons, and particularly the juice of the fruit, have so much more to offer than just slicing and dropping into a glass of gin and tonic.

Despite having a somewhat sour taste, lemons are incredibly good for us because they are packed full of Vitamin C, healthy nutrients and fibre. In fact every part of the lemon has something to offer; there are organic acids and lemon oil in the peel, fibre and antioxidants in the pith, antioxidants, vitamins, acids, minerals and lemon oil in the pulp, and salts and limonin in the pips.

The term 'superfood' has been bandied around and, as trends change, various fruits and vegetables are lauded as the next best thing. The humble lemon, however, is consistently unique in its versatility.

Nutrients

Lemons are one of the best sources of Vitamin C and just one lemon a day would provide us with our daily requirement of this nutrient. In addition lemons also contain small amounts of Vitamins B and E, as well small amounts of protein and fats. A medium-sized lemon only contains a tiny amount of sugar, just fifteen calories, plus a number of minerals, including calcium, copper, iron, manganese, magnesium, potassium, phosphorus, selenium and zinc.

In the lemon's fibre there is cellulose that helps absorb water, so it is an excellent diuretic and perfect to deal with constipation and diarrhoea. The pectin in the fibre is particularly effective in helping our bodies absorb calcium, reduce the absorption of cholesterol and suppress its production. The antioxidants in a lemon help prevent our cholesterol and body fats from being oxidized by free radicals in the body. Oxidized fats can age the skin, make us more prone to sunburn and infections, allow the formation of gall stones, give us high blood pressure and affect our eyesight. The lemon is also the only one of the citrus fruits that is capable of protecting our DNA from damage because of its high Vitamin C content.

Beauty Benefits

Every single part of a lemon contains something that can help us in our beauty regime too. We can use the juice to lighten our hair, and moisturise or cleanse our skin. Our nails

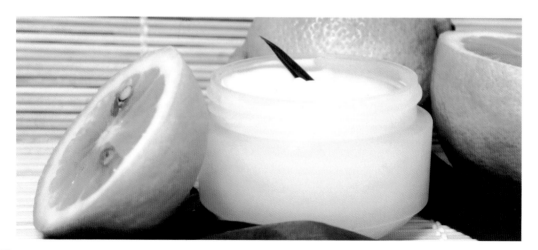

will benefit from a soak in lemon juice, too. Lemons are also present in massage oils, moisturizers, toners, deodorisers, cleansers and exfoliators.

Invaluable Household Tool

It is not just the health benefits that makes the lemon such an amazing fruit. Lemons are incredibly useful for many household chores too; from freshening the air to cleaning and polishing, to disinfection and stain removal and even dealing with annoying insects. Combining the lemon or its juice with other simple household standbys such as bicarbonate of soda (baking soda) or salt provides an inexpensive and effective cleaning product.

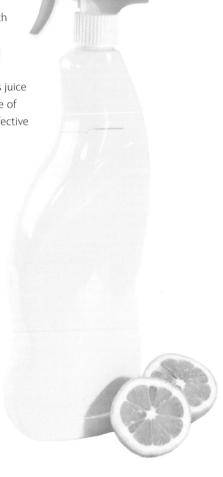

That Lemony Smell

Lemons have an unmistakeable scent and their distinctive taste comes from the acids they contain. Several other plants have a similar scent, such as lemongrass, lemon verbena or lemon balm and there are also lemon-scented varieties of popular herbs, such as mint, basil and thyme.

We are not just content to use the physical properties of the lemon, but also to make full use of the aroma they provide. That's why the lemon is such a popular additive to so many off-the-shelf cleaning products. There is something unmistakeable, fresh, clean and very appealing about that lemony smell.

All About Lemons

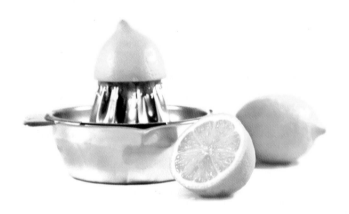

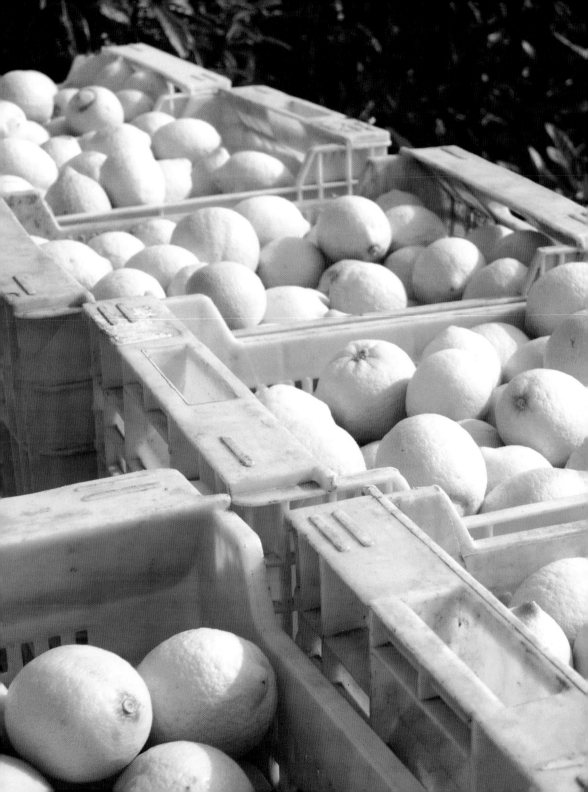

What Makes up a Lemon?

The shape and colour of the lemon makes it distinguishable from other citrus fruits – orange, grapefruit and lime. The fruit of the lemon tree starts life as a dainty, white flower, popular for bridal bouquets because of its pure white appearance. The lemon's pigment is contained in the peel and as the fruit ripens it changes from green to a vibrant yellow. All parts of the lemon contain substances beneficial to your health, in fact more so than virtually all other fruits.

Structure & Elements

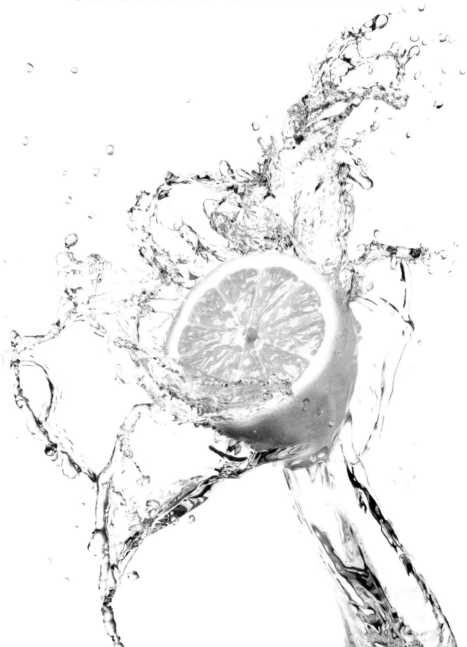

Layers

The lemon's structure consists of four main parts – peel, pith, pulp and pips. The peel, which is also known as the zest, is the shiny yellow outer layer of the lemon that can vary in thickness depending on the variety. The pith is the white, fibrous inner lining of the peel and the pulp is the segmented inside of the fruit, which produces the juice. The bitter pips are the white seeds contained within the pulp.

Dietary Fibre

The peel, pith, pips and pulp all contain dietary fibre. This is also known as roughage and can be cellulose fibre or pectin. The cellulose fibre helps the body to prevent constipation or diarrhoea by absorbing water during the digestive process. Pectin, which is also an antioxidant, encourages good bacteria in the bowel, aids the absorption of calcium, encourages the absorption of cholesterol and can help eliminate the cells that form bowel cancer.

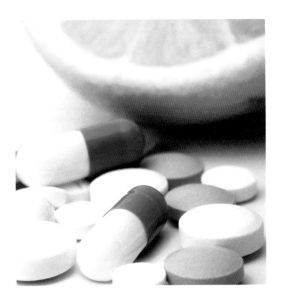

Antioxidants and Nutrients

The ascorbic acid contained in lemons makes them an excellent source of Vitamin C, an essential nutrient required for healthy formation of bones, blood vessels and skin. Even a small lemon can contain sufficient ascorbic acid to provide our daily requirement. The Vitamin C, as well as calcium, are in the juice, which should be freshly squeezed to preserve the effectiveness of the nutrients. We need antioxidants to prevent body fats, such as cholesterol, from being damaged by harmful oxidants. The peel and the pith contain the valuable nutrient iron.

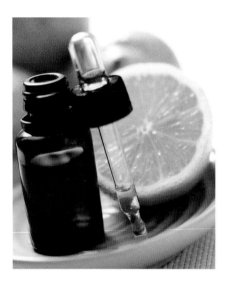

Lemon Oil

Lemon oil is extracted from the peel of the lemon and smells very 'lemony'. It is used as an essential oil and can be mixed with other oils to produce a large number of beauty and household cleaning products. Lemon oil also has health benefits because it has antibacterial, antiviral and antifungal properties, as well as being an anti-inflammatory. Lemon oil is used in conjunction with other oils in aromatherapy and is said to be soothing and relaxing. It can also improve concentration and has sedative properties.

Lemon Acids

Unlike many other fruits, lemons contain very little sugar, so they are not sweet – the bitter or sour taste of the lemon comes from its various acids. Most of the lemon acids, mainly ascorbic acid, citric acid and glucaric acid, are contained in the juice.

We have seen how essential ascorbic acid is. Citric acid helps the skin to retain water and also helps the body to move excess water from the tissues into the bloodstream, enabling the free flow of the blood supply. Glucaric acid is said to have cancer-prevention properties for a number of different cancers, including bowel, breast, prostate and colon cancer. This acid also helps lower the bad cholesterol without affecting the good cholesterol in our bodies and can prevent pre-menstrual syndrome.

The History of Lemons

There are about fifty different species of the lemon tree, which has been cultivated for around 2,500 years. It began in Asia when the lemon became popular for its antiseptic qualities and was used as an antidote for some poisons. Over the centuries the lemon tree was introduced to Europe, particularly during Roman times, then to the Arab states, followed by the Americas during the late fifteenth century. In the beginning the tree was used ornamentally, but by the eighteenth century its culinary properties began to be appreciated.

In the Beginning

Tropical Asia

The lemons cultivated in tropical Asia were probably much smaller, with thicker rinds, than those we are familiar with today. In fact lemons were not particularly popular to begin with and were often associated with superstitious beliefs. Lemons were not considered to have health benefits in the early years and it was inappropriate for children, nursing mothers or the elderly to consume them. Although the Romans painted lemons on their mosaics, it is unclear as to whether they cultivated or used the fruit.

Christopher Columbus

After becoming established in Iraq, China and the Middle East by the twelfth century and in Europe by the fifteenth century, it was Christopher Columbus who took the seeds of the lemon to America, transporting them from Europe to the New World in 1493. Lemons, together with

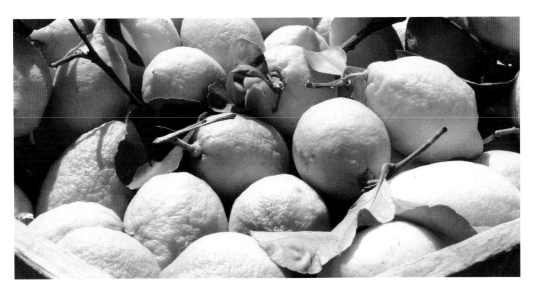

other Vitamin C fruits, became important to the miners involved in the California Gold Rush (1848–55) as a prevention of scurvy. This had also been the case in 1747, when naval surgeon James Lind had administered lemons and oranges to sailors suffering from scurvy.

Admiralty Orders

In 1795, following the work of James Lind, the British Admiralty ordered all ships to be supplied with citrus fruit – enough for each sailor to be issued with an ounce each day. On Lind's recommendation, all ships were supplied with lemon juice as their means of Vitamin C supplement. It had a dramatic effect; the health of those sailors who were given the juice was much improved compared to those who had not had it issued.

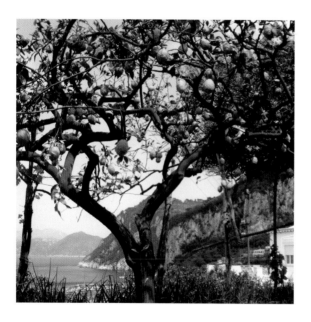

The Lemon Spreads

The Dutch introduced the lemon tree to South Africa and the English introduced the fruit to Australia towards the end of the eighteenth century. Within a hundred years the fruit was being grown in large quantities in the United States, as well as in many Mediterranean countries with a sub-tropical climate. Now around a quarter of all lemon trees grown in the world are in California, with the other major lemon producers being Argentina, Greece, Italy, Spain and Turkey.

Why a Sub-Tropical Climate?

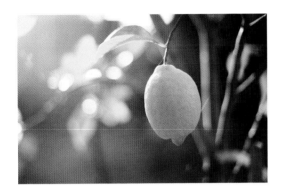

Bring Me Sunshine

Because lemon trees need warmth and sunshine they thrive in sub-tropical climates, although they can be grown in a greenhouse or conservatory in countries that do not have the benefit of warm weather conditions. Ideal growing conditions require good drainage, so a gently sloping site is often chosen. Bees pollinate the flowers of the lemon tree and this encourages the fruit to form, so a wind-free situation is ideal, as the bee has the opportunity to rest and pollinate. Mulching, regular feeding and pruning all help maintain the lemon tree in prime condition to bear plentiful amounts of fruit. Watering is of prime importance if the tree is to bear succulent, juicy fruit.

Harvesting Lemons

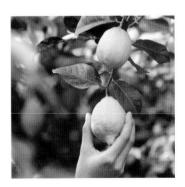

In sub-tropical climates the lemon tree can be harvested several times a year. This is unlike many other citrus trees, which tend to only flower in winter and spring. When the fruit is ready to be picked it is cut off at the stem, just above the fruit, and left unwashed. This helps to preserve the lemons and protects them from becoming susceptible to mould and mildew.

Sourcing & Using Lemons

If you do not live in a sub-tropical climate then the chances are you will have to rely on your local greengrocer or supermarket to source your lemons. Sadly, you will not experience the delight of plucking one from a tree, but that does not mean you cannot have some simple tactics for choosing the best available. With more than 13 million tonnes of lemons being produced worldwide every year, you should be able to source some decent ones.

Be Picky!

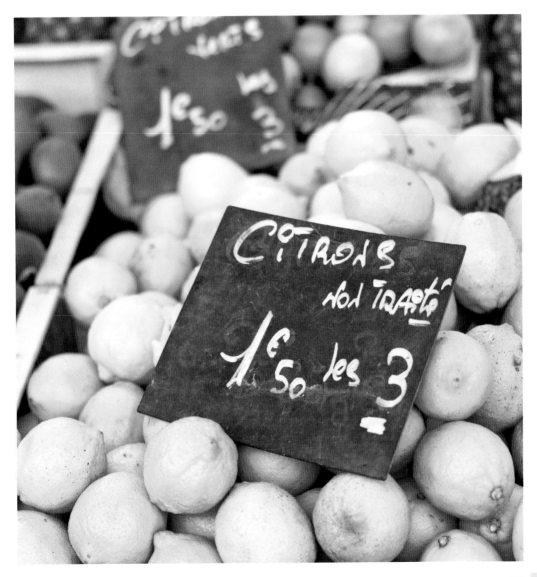

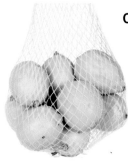

Only the Best Will Do

Whether you buy lemons at a market stall, a greengrocer or a large supermarket, you should feel the fruit you are going to buy. Opt for smooth skins because this usually means less peel and more pulp, which means more juice. Sometimes you can tell by the weight; if the lemon is small but quite heavy then it should be full of pulp and juice. Ignore any fruit that has blemishes, or is shrivelled or spongy when gently squeezed in the palm of the hand.

Colour and Appearance

Choose a deep yellow colour lemon that is firm to the touch (but not too hard), not too large at each end and shows no sign of damage. Bruised or damaged lemons will not keep as well because they will be susceptible to mould. A good-quality lemon should feel oily but fine and smooth-skinned.

Waxed or Unwaxed?

With any number of pesticides, fungicides, insecticides, bactericides and preservatives being sprayed during the growing process, the best option is to choose an organic unwaxed lemon. This is particularly important if you intend to use the lemon peel, as normally organic and unwaxed lemons have had no routine use of pesticides at any stage of the growing or transportation process. This helps to ensure that the peel is untreated and that no pesticide or wax has penetrated the pulp of the lemon. If you are unsure about whether or not the lemon has been waxed, or what it may have been treated with, then washing it well before use will at least remove any substance that has remained on the peel.

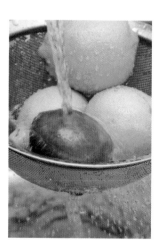

Storing Your Lemons

In the Refrigerator

Whole lemons can be kept in a plastic bag in the refrigerator for up to 10 days, or perhaps even longer. It will start to shrivel when it is no longer fresh and the skin of the fruit will take on a pitted look. If you do not have a refrigerator then a cool, dark room is a good substitute.

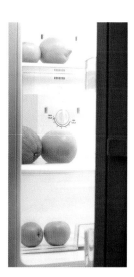

Freezing

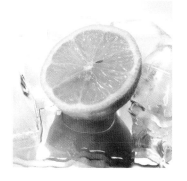

Do not be tempted to freeze a whole lemon, as once it thaws it will probably only be useful for puree, or at best to be chopped. You can freeze the juice and the zest, though. Try filling ice-cube trays with juice so you freeze it with recipe-sized portions. Or to give your ice-cubes a bit of a tangy kick, add a few drops of lemon juice to the water before freezing.

Strips, Peels and Wedges

Lemon peel can also be stored in a refrigerator in an airtight bag for several days. Or strips of peel can be frozen, as can slices of lemon, or lemon wedges. If you want to store lemon wedges for a few days then cover them in clingfilm. However if you are saving the lemon wedges for a savoury dish, you can preserve them for a few days by coating them in vinegar.

Using Your Lemons

It's All in the Preparation!

If you are using a waxed lemon for cooking, it is advisable to wash it in hot, clean, washing-up water before beginning your preparation. This is to remove any pesticides that may have been sprayed on the fruit to help preserve it. Alternatively you could boil a kettle and fill a basin with the hot water, then submerge the lemon(s) for 30 seconds to dissolve the wax. Whichever method you use, remember to rinse the lemon under cold, running water before beginning your preparation.

Juicing a Lemon

To get the most juice possible out of a stored lemon, remove the fruit from the refrigerator in good time. A lemon at room temperature will provide you with much more juice than one that has been kept cold in the refrigerator. A medium-sized lemon should provide 2–3 tbsp/30–45ml/1–1½ fl oz of juice.

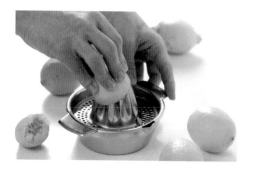

Another tip is to either pop the lemon in the microwave for 10 to 15 seconds, or roll the lemon with your hand on the work surface. Both of these methods help produce more lemon juice, as the pulp's membranes are broken down.

You can squeeze the lemon to obtain juice in a number of different ways. You could use your hands, provided they are big enough and strong enough. Manual lemon squeezers come in glass, metal or plastic. These have a ribbed top and a tray to catch the pips, with a collecting area for the juice you've managed to extract. There are also electric versions of this type of citrus squeezer.

You can also buy a 'citrus reamer', which is a wooden, metal or plastic hand-held version of the classic squeezer – you push the conical end into the lemon half and grind out the juice. Then there are also wooden or metal, hand-held lemon squeezers that are often called 'citrus trumpets'. The ribbed top is screwed into the lemon and rotated to obtain the juice, which pours out of the trumpet-shaped end.

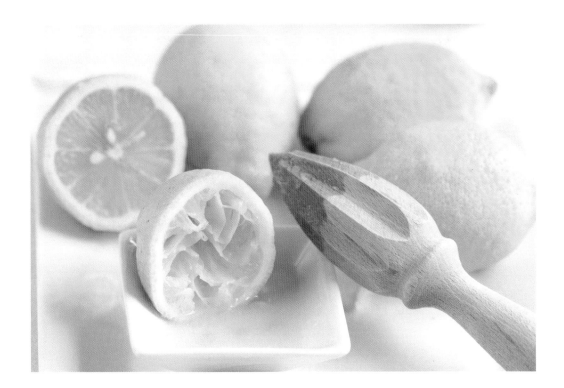

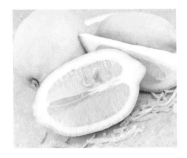

Wedges

The term 'lemon wedges' relates to chunks of lemon, or a lemon that has been cut into four quarters. Often these are used to accompany fish, meat or vegetable dishes and are squeezed at the table, or they are added to drinks. When being used with food, the shape of the wedge helps eliminate the juice spraying everywhere when the lemon is squeezed.

To produce the perfect wedge you should first cut the lemon in half lengthways. It is important to cut off the pointed section of each end of the lemon at this stage to square the lemon off and give it a more tailored appearance. Try not to remove any of the flesh of the lemon, but just remove the protruding ends. Then remove any of the white pith that accumulates in the centre of the pulp with a sharp knife. Take out obvious pips too if you can. Now divide each half of the lemon into two wedges, or three pieces if the lemon is a particularly large one. You can prepare the wedges in advance of serving your meal and you can store them in the refrigerator, covered in clingfilm to retain their juice.

Muddling, Slicing and Twisting

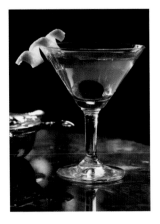

Muddling a citrus fruit involves using a pestle to press down on the lemon or lime. This crushes the fruit, releasing the juice and some of the oils that are contained in the zest or peel. To muddle a lemon you should cut it in half and then cut each of the halves into quarters. This provides the wedges of fruit ready to be pressed. Using the pestle, press down until all the juice has been extracted.

To prepare lemon slices, you should cut the lemon in half lengthways and lay the fruit on a chopping board with the fruit side facing down. Cut across the lemon with a sharp knife and create slices about 5 mm (⅕ inch) thick.

A lemon twist is also used when serving drinks, particularly cocktails. Cut the ends off the lemon and remove the pulp using a spoon. Keep this pulp, as it can be stored in the refrigerator for later use. Slice the lemon peel lengthwise into strips of about 6 mm (¼ inch) thick. As the drink is being served, rub the inside of the glass with the lemon peel and then twist the strip of peel like a corkscrew. Serve the twist on the rim of the glass, or drop it into the drink.

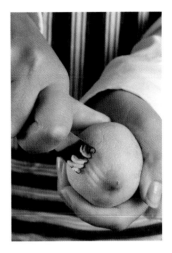

Lemon Zest

The zest of a lemon refers only to the bright yellow peel and not the white pith that lines it. The pith is very bitter, although it does have some nutrient value. Zest has a very strong lemon flavour and is an ideal flavouring for many recipes.

You can grate the peel using a conventional grater, but choose the finest option and brush the zest off with a pastry brush. A traditional lemon zester can also be used. This cuts long, thin, threadlike strands of zest through its tiny cutting holes. If you do not have a zester or grater, use a vegetable peeler or a small, sharp, paring knife. Carefully peel off a strip of the lemon zest, making sure you only take the yellow layer. If there is any pith showing on the underside of the peel then it is best to remove this.

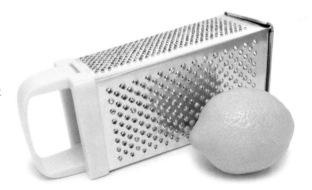

Cleaning & Laundry

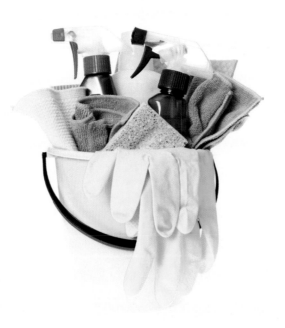

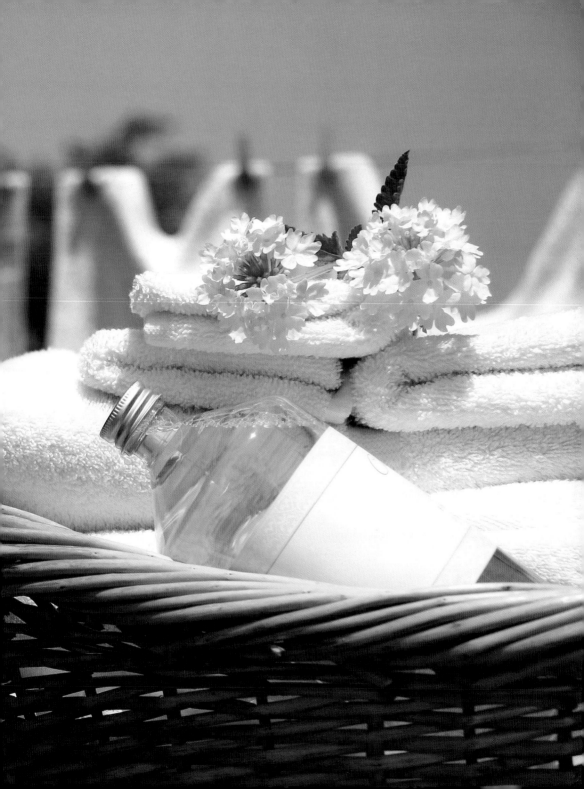

Cleaning Around the House

Most detergents and general household cleaning products are expensive and packed with chemicals. The humble lemon is a natural, organic, environmentally friendly, perfect substitute for many of these harmful household cleaning products. Lemons are an incredibly useful cleaning resource and they can be used for a huge variety of different chores in the home. They cost just a fraction of the price and are so much better for your health. And they smell terrific!

All-Purpose Cleaning Solutions

Mineral and Limescale Build-up

Lemons are great for removing the build-up of limescale from around stainless steel sinks and draining boards. The lemon peel is also excellent at keeping chrome taps free from limescale. All you have to do is cut a lemon in half and rub it over the affected area. Leave the lemon to do its work for at least a minute and then rinse with cold water and buff with a soft, dry cloth.

CAUTION: Do not use lemon juice or the peel on gold-plated taps and plug holes as this can cause them to tarnish.

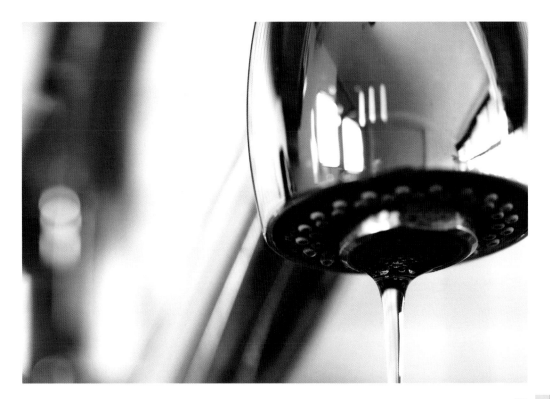

Disinfectant

If you want to kill bacteria without having to clean off the residue left by most chemical cleaning products, why not use a lemon? The acids contained in lemon juice kill off the bacteria, which do not survive long in an acidic environment. Lemon juice can disinfect most kitchen worktops, including chopping boards and sinks, as well as bathroom sinks and surfaces. The juice kills the bacteria in a natural way and leaves a fresh fragrance.

Why not try adding a small amount of lemon juice to drinking water to ensure that no bacteria are surviving there?

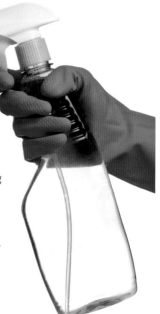

Degreaser

Pure lemon juice is a great way to get rid of a grease build-up. You have to apply the juice liberally to the affected area and give it a little time to cut through the grease, but it does work and you also have the added bonus of the fresh smell of lemons. The limonene in the lemon's essential oil is what removes the grease and this also has anti-bacterial properties.

Furnishings & Surfaces

Tarnished Copper, Aluminium and Brass Pans

You know how pots and pans can get tarnished so quickly, particularly copper-bottomed ones? Well, it is not necessary to stand and polish them for hours with a proprietary product

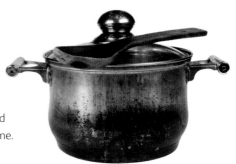

if you've got lemons and salt to hand. In fact it isn't restricted to just salt, as you could also dip half a lemon into some bicarbonate of soda (baking soda). Salt and bicarbonate of soda are mild abrasives and the acid in the lemon dissolves the tarnish. Rinse with cold water and buff with a dry, soft cloth to bring back the shine.

You can also make a paste to coat a badly tarnished copper or brass pan. Mix together 50 ml/2 fl oz/¼ cup of ordinary table salt and moisten it with enough lemon juice to make a firm paste. Leave the mix for 10 minutes and then spread it onto your tarnished pots and pans. Then just rinse the item in ordinary, warm tap water and dry with a clean, dry cloth. You can repeat this any number of times without damaging the pot.

Silver and Brass Polish

Whether you want to preserve ornaments or grandma's best cutlery, lemon juice and bicarbonate of soda (baking soda) will help to keep them shiny. Mix the lemon juice and soda into a thick paste and rub it into the silver or brass with a soft cloth. Give it five minutes to work and then wash the ornament or cutlery well in warm water and washing-up liquid.

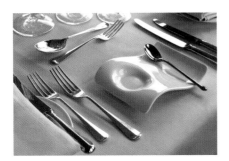

Another remedy that originated in Greece for cleaning silver cutlery is to mix together lemon juice and neat washing-up liquid. Apply the mix directly to the piece of cutlery with a soft cloth and then rinse off and buff with a clean, dry cloth.

CAUTION: Do not leave the paste on your best silver for too long or the acid in the lemon juice could cause pitting.

Furniture Polish

The limonene in the lemon's essential oils can dissolve the different types of grime that build up on wooden furniture. This can include old furniture polish, wax, fingerprints and general dust and dirt. To make your own furniture polish, mix together, in a sealable container so it will keep, 250 ml/8 fl oz/1 cup of olive oil with 120 ml/4 fl oz/½ cup of freshly squeezed and strained lemon juice. You need to strain the lemon juice before mixing it with the olive oil to make sure there are no residual lumps of lemon pulp. Now dab a little of your mixture onto a clean cloth and polish the furniture in the normal way. The lemon juice is great for grime-busting, but the olive oil also gives wooden furniture a lovely shine and nourishes the wood, too. This mixture can also be used for bringing a shine to hardwood floors.

Guitar Cleaner

Most stringed instruments can be cleaned effectively with lemon. The lemon oil is efficient in stripping off the grime build-up and you can even get into all those grooves and crevices.

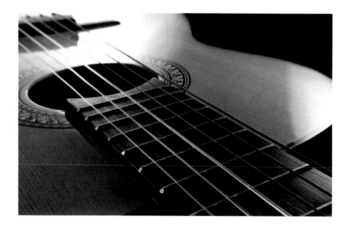

CAUTION: Do not use this remedy on guitars that are made from maple wood, as they are sealed with a varnish or lacquer coating, which prevents dirt and grime from getting into the pores of the wood and accumulating.

Windows and Mirrors

Wedges of lemon can be rubbed over windows and mirrors to effectively clean and shine them. Squeeze the wedge of lemon as you rub to release some of the lemon juice then wipe the glass with a dampened cloth immediately. Then buff with a clean, dry cloth to produce the shine.

Glass and China

To remove the build-up of limescale that can accumulate on china and drinking glasses, make a solution of water and lemon juice. Use the two ingredients in equal quantities and let this solution sit in the cup or glass for several hours. Then wash up as normal in hot water and washing-up liquid. This remedy also helps remove stubborn stains that build up in cups from tea and coffee.

It Works on all Floor Types

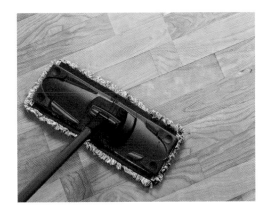

Most types of floors can be cleaned effectively by combining lemon oil with other natural products. For a simple mix, add 4 tbsp of white vinegar to a bucket of hot water. Then add 10 drops of lemon oil before mopping the floor as normal.

Ceramic tiled floors, as well as hardwood and laminate floors, can also be cleaned using a combination of lemon oil, water, white vinegar and your own choice of two more essential oils, for example tea-tree oil and lavender, geranium or bergamot. To create this great-smelling and effective floor cleaner, mix together 250 ml/8 fl oz/1 cup of both white vinegar and water. Then add five drops each of the lemon oil and your choice of two other essential oils. You can use a spray bottle to lightly apply the mixture to the floor before mopping or wiping with a clean, preferably lint-free cloth.

Metal Cleaner

You can clean metal by first dissolving some salt in hot lemon juice (for the juice of one lemon use one tablespoon of salt) and then applying the mixture with a cloth to the item. Rinse well and dry with a clean, soft cloth.

Alternatively, soak a clean cloth in lemon juice and then dip it into some salt before rubbing on the metal. Or if you don't want to use a cloth, you can cut a lemon in half before dipping it into the salt and applying it directly to the metal item. Whichever method you choose, make sure you rinse the item well and then dry with a clean cloth.

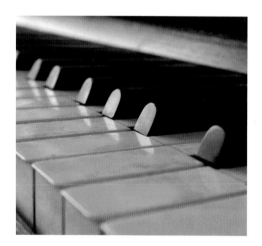

Marble and Ivory Surfaces Cleaner

If you have marble worktops, or marble-topped pieces of furniture, you will know that they can become stained and how hard it is to remove those stains. If you cut a lemon in half and dip it in some salt you can use this to scrub the stain. Make sure you rinse the lemon juice off the surface thoroughly, though.

The same applies to ivory surfaces, such as piano keys or knife handles. To whiten ivory piano keys or knife handles that have yellowed, try rubbing them with lemon juice that has been diluted with an equal amount of water. Apply this mix carefully so that none of the liquid gets into the metal parts of the piano, then wipe dry with a clean, soft cloth.

CAUTION: Antique piano keys are often made of ivory and this naturally reacts to the environment, so trying to remove the yellowing may reduce the antique-look and therefore possibly the value of the piano as a whole.

Odour Removal from Wooden Surfaces

Wooden surfaces, like kitchen worktops and chopping boards, can harbour harmful germs and soak up a variety of different food odours. Onions, fish and garlic are good examples of foods that can soak into wood and stay there. Rub half a lemon liberally over the wooden surface. Let the lemon juice dry fully, then rinse it off with cold water. This will disinfect the surface and remove all those unpleasant odours.

Wooden furniture can also harbour smells, such as pet 'deposits' and stale tobacco. Rubbing with half a lemon can help remove the odours.

If your wooden furniture has drawers, then try placing a small dish of bicarbonate of soda (baking soda) mixed with lemon juice inside the drawer. This will help to neutralize any lingering smells.

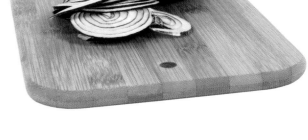

CAUTION: Do not use this odour-beating remedy on highly polished wooden furniture as the lemon may be too acidic.

Kitchen & Bathroom

Our kitchens and bathrooms can harbour any number of unpleasant bacteria and odours. Because lemons are so good at disinfecting, cleaning and removing lingering smells, they are the ideal, natural way to keep kitchen appliances and bathroom surfaces fresh and germ free. Lemons work just as well as expensive chemicals and they are much kinder to the household, its inhabitants and the environment in general. Read on and see what lemons can do for refrigerators, dishwashers and other appliances and utensils.

Kitchen Appliances

Dishwasher Cleaner

Although you can buy dishwasher fresheners and cleaners, using half a lemon gives just as good a result. Cut the lemon in half and impale it onto one of the upright prongs inside the dishwasher. The acid in the lemon will degrease the appliance and the fresh lemon smell will linger for several cycles.

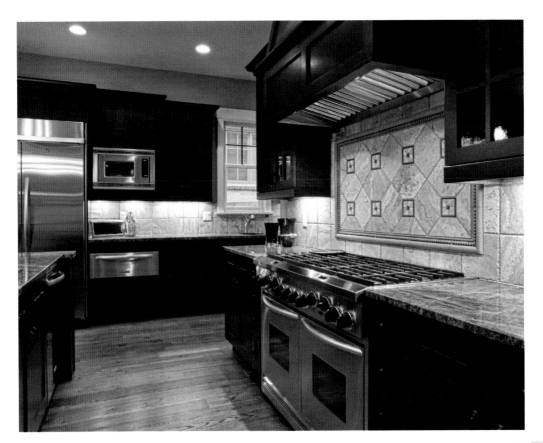

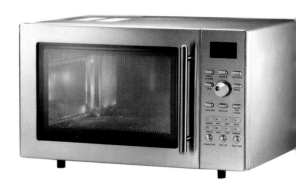

Microwave Cleaner

Stale food smells can linger for ages in a microwave and they seem to be accentuated each time you use the appliance. Placing one or two slices of lemon in a cup of water and running the microwave on high for 30 seconds will really help clean it. The lemon will be steamed in the microwave and all that is required is a clean, dry cloth to wipe away the excess steam.

An alternative way of effectively freshening up the microwave is to make a paste using 1 tsp of white vinegar, 50 ml/2 fl oz/¼ cup of bicarbonate of soda (baking soda) and 6 drops of lemon oil. Simply apply this paste to the inside surfaces of the microwave and then rinse with cold water. If you leave the door of the microwave open for a while then the air will help to dry your clean and bacteria-free microwave.

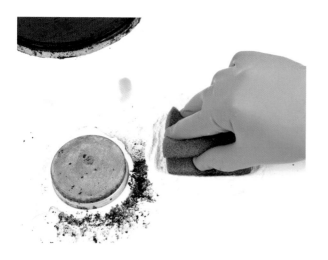

Stove-top Spills

Lemon juice is well known for its natural cleaning powers, but when mixed with bicarbonate of soda (baking soda) it is a potent mix. Mix together some bicarbonate of soda, lemon juice and warm water and spread this paste over the stove top or hob spill. The bicarbonate of soda (baking soda) is a mild abrasive and the lemon juice has great degreasing properties. Rinse well to make sure the surface does not remain powdery and buff dry with a clean cloth.

Oven Cleaner

You can use the bicarbonate of soda (baking soda) and lemon juice mix inside the oven too. Because lemons contain natural lemon oil and acid they boost the cleaning process by dissolving grease.

Make sure the oven is completely cool before you apply the lemony bicarbonate of soda (baking soda) paste. Good proportions to make the ideal paste are 2 tbsp of bicarbonate of soda (baking soda) to 250 ml/8 fl oz/1 cup of water. To this mix add the juice of a whole lemon. You'll have a clean oven and a fresh smelling kitchen too.

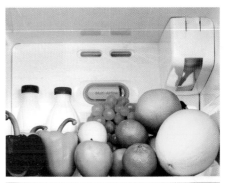

Refrigerator Odour Reducer

Even if you haven't mistakenly left food in the refrigerator and it has gone bad, fridges can still get very smelly. Every time you open the door you'll probably notice it. If you place half a lemon in a small dish at the back of the fridge this can really help as the lemon absorbs the smell for a good length of time. So when you have to put your head into the fridge to clean it, the job won't seem quite so distasteful.

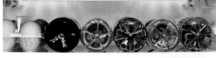

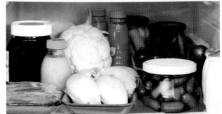

Surfaces & Utensils

Kitchen Cabinet Cleaner

Sticky, greasy fingers are usually the culprits when our kitchen cabinet doors look messy. To get rid of the grease and make your cabinets look like new, just make a solution of lemon juice and hot water. Use about 50 ml/2 fl oz/¼ cup of freshly squeezed lemon juice and 250 ml/8 fl oz/1 cup of hot water. Stir the solution and simply wipe onto your cabinets with a clean cloth.

Sink Cleaner

Because lemons have a mild bleaching property they are great for removing stains on kitchen and bathroom sinks. As well as being a bleaching agent, lemon is also capable of dissolving soap scum and limescale, and it disinfects into the bargain. So there are several handy uses in one natural product.

It is the acid in the lemon that is very effective in getting rid of soap scum build-up. Use neat lemon juice and a sponge to coat the soap scum. Leave it for a few hours to do its work and then rinse with cold water.

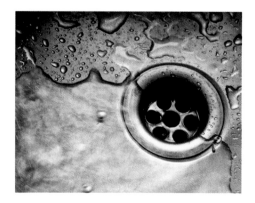

Rub half a lemon over your draining boards and taps, then rinse and dry with a clean cloth. This will disinfect and break down any limescale build-up. Lemon juice is a great way to rid your kitchen of a smelly sink!

If your sink has a waste or garbage disposal unit installed you can keep it smelling fresh using lemon peel. Put lemon peel through the unit regularly and rinse with water. It's as easy as that!

Clean Dirty Dishes

If your dishes need a really good scrub, don't reach for the pan scourers, reach for a lemon. Make a paste with lemon juice, white vinegar and bicarbonate of soda (baking soda) to scour away the stains on your dishes. Use 1 tsp of white vinegar, 50 ml/2 fl oz/¼ cup of bicarbonate of soda (baking soda) and squeeze in the juice of half a lemon to scrub away those stains.

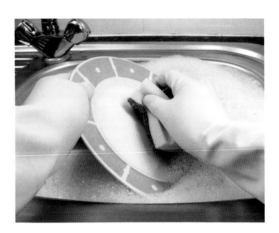

Alternatively, dip half a lemon into bicarbonate of soda (baking soda) and use this to do the scouring. It is equally effective at removing stains from dishes. Although with a little forethought you could pour neat lemon juice onto any baked-on stain and let the dish soak for 10 or 15 minutes. When you come to wash the dish it will be much easier, as the acid in the lemon will have helped to dissolve the baked-on stain. Then you probably won't need to scrub at all!

Clean Discoloured Kitchen Utensils

Stainless steel, wooden or plastic kitchen utensils can all benefit from the lemon treatment. Wooden and plastic ones in particular can become discoloured and stained. Use the paste you used to clean the dirty dishes to clean them too.

To buff up stainless steel utensils use neat lemon juice mixed with a little salt as your polishing agent. Apply the mixture liberally and then rinse off before buffing with a clean, dry cloth. You'll be amazed at how shiny the lemon juice makes your kitchen utensils look.

Clean Discoloured Plastic Containers

Lemons and the sun are the answer for making your discoloured plastic boxes and containers look like new. If your plastic boxes have become discoloured inside then rub half a lemon over their inside surface. Make sure you do this on a nice sunny day and let the container sit in full sunlight for as long as possible. The lemon's mild bleaching properties combined with the sun's ability to whiten make this combination a really effective stain remover. You can use it on plastic kitchen utensils, too.

Remove Soft Cheese or Sticky Foods from a Grater

Do you ever use recipes that involve grating sticky foods, such as soft cheese, and you have to try to poke out all the bits that are stuck in the holes of the grater? Well, lemon pulp is the answer. Rub half a lemon over both sides of the grater when you've finished preparing your food and this will easily get rid of the residue. Rinse it when you've finished to watch the bits float away down the plughole.

Remove Fruit and Berry Stains from Hands

So you've all been fruit-picking and you've just arrived home. Everyone has purple hands, they are eager to eat and they begin to sit on your cream sofas. Soap and hot water often

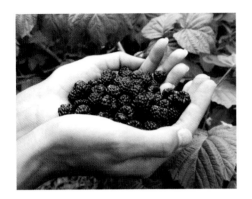

do not remove those fruit and berry stains from the hands, but neat lemon juice will. Squeeze lemon juice onto your hands and rub them together for a few minutes before you wash them with soap and water. The lemon juice lifts the stains much easier than soap alone.

Of course you can clean your hands in the same way if they become stained whilst you are preparing your berries for your recipe.

Remove Berry Stains from Your Worktops, Too!

If any berry juice dribbles onto your kitchen work surface lemon juice will remove those stains, too. Pour some freshly squeezed lemon juice onto the stain, then sprinkle some bicarbonate of soda (baking soda) over it. Let this combination do its job for about an hour before gently scrubbing the stain. Then you can rinse the clean work surface.

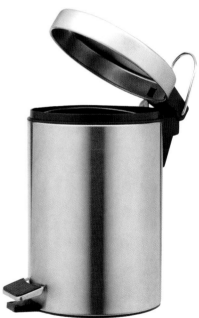

Don't Forget the Kitchen Bin!

We've all got one, whether it is metal or plastic. We replace bin liners, and wash the bin frequently, but somehow they still seem to harbour a smell of their own. Why not try putting some lemon peel in the bottom of your bin – it really does help rid your kitchen of that bin smell.

Bathroom

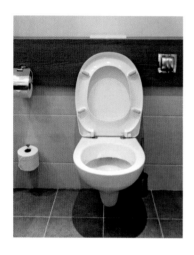

Toilet-bowl Cleaner

Because lemons are acidic they are excellent anti-bacterial and antiseptic cleaning products. We all know that bleach can easily ruin clothes if you are unfortunate enough to splash some on yourself when cleaning the toilet.

Bicarbonate of soda (baking soda), white vinegar and lemon juice are a perfect replacement for those other harsh, caustic chemicals. Sprinkle some bicarbonate of soda (baking soda) into the toilet bowl and leave it for about half an hour before scrubbing with a toilet brush and flushing.

You can remove more stubborn toilet stains, like a build-up of limescale, by sprinkling in the bicarbonate of soda (baking soda) and then pouring a dash of white vinegar mixed with lemon juice. The white vinegar doesn't smell that good on its own, but adding the lemon juice gives your toilet a lovely fresh smell.

Toilet Seats

You can use bicarbonate of soda (baking soda) on any kind of toilet seat too to get rid of stains. If you add a little lemon juice to the soda the solution will also freshen up the whole bathroom. When you've finished wiping the upper and lower sides of the toilet seat you can flush the solution down the loo for a really thorough clean.

Soap and Scum Removal

We all get soap scum in our bath, shower and sink. It is that horrible white or pale-grey layer that builds up as a result of hard water. When the hard water gets mixed with soap and household dust it can become difficult to get remove.

Use 2 tbsp of lemon juice mixed with 900 ml/1½ pints/3¾ cups of very hot water to help remove the scum. Use a spray bottle to coat the layers of soap scum and let the mixture do its job for about 10 minutes before wiping it off with a clean, damp cloth. The acid in the lemon juice cuts through soap scum. The solution works equally well on tiles, shower cubicles, sinks or work surfaces. They will all look shiny and the whole bathroom will smell good.

If necessary you can apply neat lemon juice directly onto a sponge or cloth and wash the affected area. Leave the lemon juice to work for a few hours before rinsing it off.

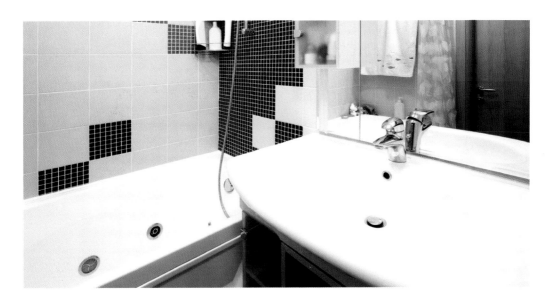

Laundry

You can see them all as you walk around the store –
stain removers, clothes' whiteners, special washing
powder or gel tabs for coloured clothes, fabric
softeners. Is it not ironic that although all of these
might work, the humble lemon is equally effective for
the majority of laundry jobs? Lemon juice can remove
the most stubborn stains, including rust and mildew,
because of its amazing bleaching properties. The
bonus is that you get sweet-smelling clothes and save
money on expensive products.

Stain & Odour Removal

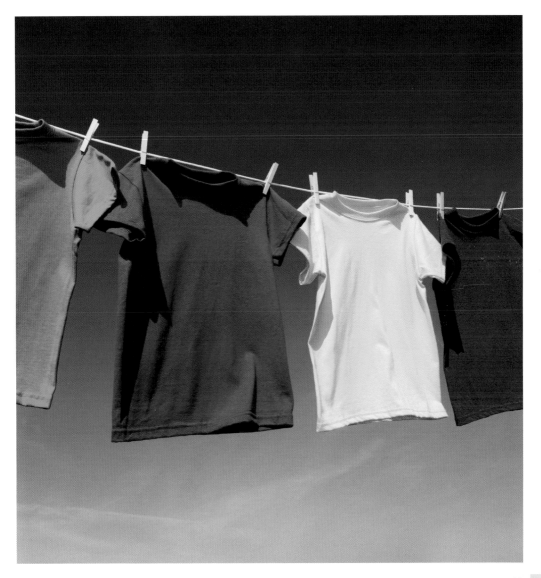

Freshen White Laundry

Some washing powders claim they wash whiter, and that it shows, but they've probably not used lemons. The bleaching effect of lemon juice can really work on keeping your whites white. Add lemon juice to your normal wash cycle. How much you pop into the washing machine will depend on the amount of white laundry you are hoping to whiten. For a complete bed set of whites use the juice of one or two lemons, but for a couple of white tops just squeeze in half a lemon.

As a Bleach or Whitener

Rather than risking the use of proprietary bleaching products to remove stains, why not try using lemons instead? The problem with using bleach is that it can actually stain clothes itself. This is because it can lift elements of iron from the water system and stain your clothing during the wash cycle.

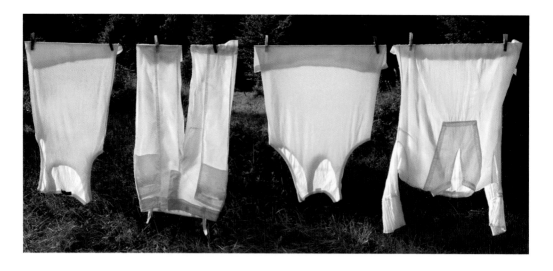

For a failsafe way of removing stains or whitening clothes, soak them in a mixture of half lemon juice and half water before washing. If the clothes are badly stained you might find it useful, in addition to the pre-soak, to add lemon juice to the washing machine too. Those stains definitely will not survive both these treatments!

Don't forget the power of the sun and lemon combined. Your whites, once pre-soaked and then washed with the added lemon juice, will dazzle if you hang them on the line on a sunny day. The sun will help bleach those stains, too!

White Sports Socks

To keep those white sports socks white and eliminate the discolouration you so often get on the bottoms of the feet, try boiling them in a pan of equal amounts of hot water and lemon juice.

Tea-stain Removal

Before you decide to dispose of that favourite top or other tea-stained item you have spilled tea over, have a go at removing the stain with lemon. As with all stains on clothing, it is wise to treat it as soon as possible for an effective removal.

If your clothing can be washed in hot water, try pouring 250 ml/8 fl oz/1 cup of lemon juice into the washing machine and wash the item straight away. If this is not possible, at the very least sprinkle some lemon juice over the tea stain. This will remove the colour from the stain. Then wash it in the machine, including the lemon juice of course, at the earliest opportunity.

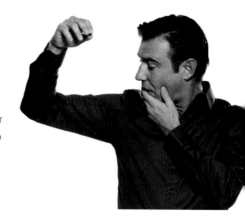

Underarm Sweat Stains

Some shirts and blouses seem to get very discoloured under the arms, especially white clothing. Mix together a potion of half lemon juice and half water, then scrub gently at the stain to remove any ugly marks.

Fruit and Fruit Juice Stain Removal

We already know that lemon juice is effective for removing berry stains from hands and kitchen work surfaces. Well, it is just as effective on removing fruit stains from clothing. It doesn't really matter what variety of fruit has found its way onto your clothes, because lemon juice works well on them all. If you sprinkle some neat lemon juice over the stain before washing it will help the stain to fade. Add more lemon juice to the washing machine and it will never survive!

Rust Stain Removal

Whatever you do, don't be tempted to put proprietary bleach onto a rust stain because all it will do is set hard. Instead, sprinkle the clothing with a generous amount of table salt. Squeeze a lemon over the salt and place the item of clothing outside in the sun. If possible keep it in direct sunlight for several hours, adding more lemon juice if the clothing begins to dry out. Before you pop it into the washing machine, with added lemon juice of course, brush the salt off what should now be a faded stain.

Scorch-mark Removal

It has happened to all of us; you're busy ironing and someone rings the doorbell or telephones and you leave the iron face down on the clothing. When you return there is a brownish, iron-shaped mark that you feel sure will never come out in the wash. If it happens again, try lemon juice. Squeeze a lemon over the stain and let it dry in direct sunlight. Timing will depend on the thickness of the fabric and the intensity of the sun. Hopefully if it hasn't actually burned the fabric, the lemon juice and sunlight combined will lighten the stain, although you may have to repeat the process to make it disappear altogether.

Mildew Stain Removal

To remove mildew stains on washable clothing you need a trusty lemon. Sprinkle the stains generously with table salt and liberally pour lemon juice over the salt. Then let that magic combination of lemon and sun remove the stain. Leave it to dry in direct sunlight for several hours, but continue to keep the area moist by adding more lemon juice periodically. Brush off the salt before putting the item in the washing machine – and don't forget you can add more lemon juice to the wash cycle too if needed.

The lemon juice will also help eliminate the smell of mildew, which can so often linger, even after washing.

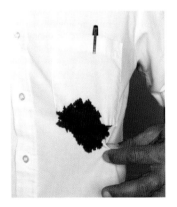

Ink-stain Removal

As with all types of staining on your clothing, it is good to remember that new stains are easier to remove than old ones. So if you spill ink on an item of clothing, the best thing to do is mop up the excess ink immediately. Then try sprinkling table salt onto the stain and generously apply neat lemon juice on top. Put the item of clothing in direct sunlight for as long as possible, moistening regularly with more lemon juice. Wash as normal, but if the stain has only lightened and not disappeared then repeat the whole process.

Colour & Condition

Keep Clothes Bright

There are a number of tips available for keeping your coloured clothes bright and to prevent them from fading, including washing inside out and hanging out to dry inside out. Another useful tip for those who like to use nature's way is to add 120 ml/4 fl oz/½ cup of white

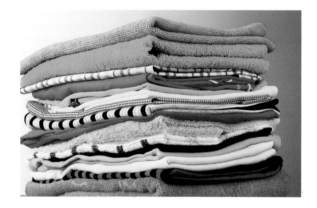

vinegar to the washing-machine. Vinegar doesn't smell good, even though it is effective for retaining the vibrancy of colour, so add a few drops of lemon juice to the vinegar before putting it into the washing machine and this really improves the smell.

CAUTION: Do not add too much lemon juice because of its bleaching properties.

Lint Removal

Some people say that vinegar works well on a piece of cloth or a sponge to remove lint build-up on clothing. Well, lemon juice works just as well. Soak the cloth or sponge in the lemon juice and dab away at the lint. The lemon juice will soak it up. Another way of using a lemon to remove the lint is to treat half a lemon like a piece of sticky tape. The fibrous pulp and pith of the lemon will grab the lint from the clothing as you dab away.

Pre-Treat Laundry Solution

Good old lemon juice can work wonders for removing stains, as we already know. It is advisable to treat all stains before washing, as they can become ground-in during the washing process. Undiluted or mixed with water, lemon juice is an excellent pre-treatment for all your laundry problems.

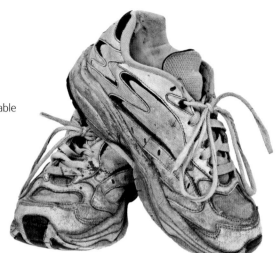

Whiten Athletic Shoes

If your tennis or canvas athletic shoes have begun to look a bit grubby, there's no need to reach for the bleach bottle to whiten them. Lemon juice will do it. Spray them with lemon juice all over – inside and out. Then place them in the direct sunlight to dry. They will be stain-free and much whiter when you return to them and they'll probably smell much better too!

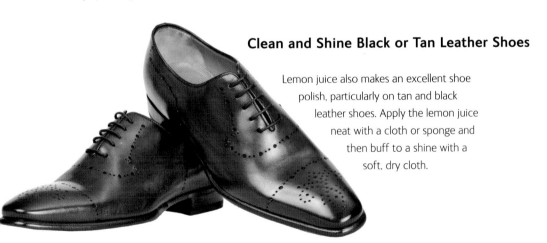

Clean and Shine Black or Tan Leather Shoes

Lemon juice also makes an excellent shoe polish, particularly on tan and black leather shoes. Apply the lemon juice neat with a cloth or sponge and then buff to a shine with a soft, dry cloth.

Home & Garden

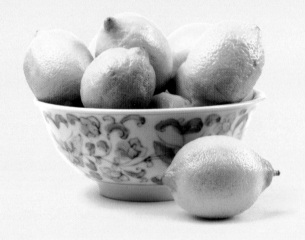

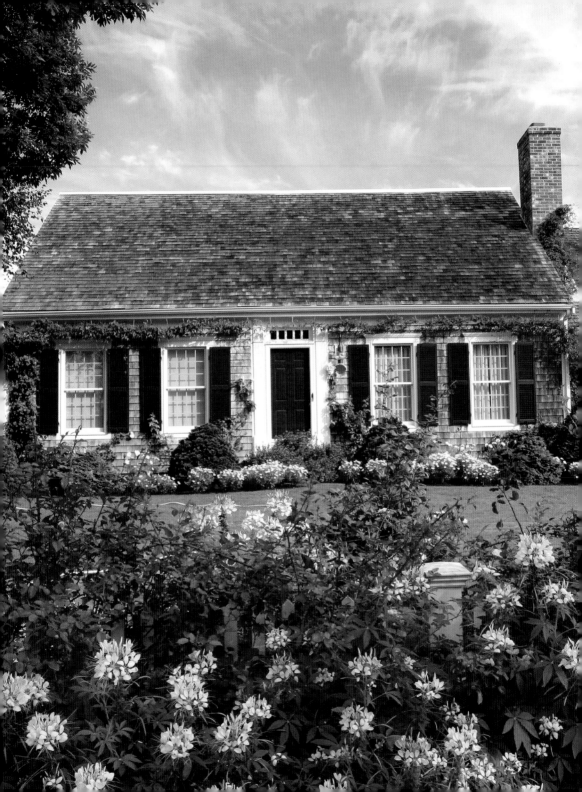

General Household

The refreshing and invigorating smell of lemons symbolizes for many a clean and well-kept home. That's why so many producers of those proprietary cleaners and fresheners add lemon to their products as a preference. But lemons do not just smell fresh; they have lots of useful, cheap and chemical-free uses around the home. Have a look and see what else lemons and their juice can do. You'll be amazed at how flexible lemons are, as well as being better for the environment.

Odour Removal

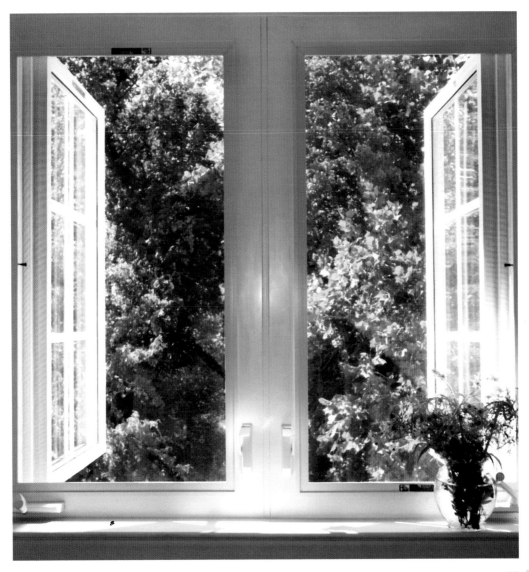

Air Freshener

To refresh the air in the kitchen, particularly if you've been cooking fish or strong-smelling foods like garlic, cut a lemon in half and immerse it in a pan of water. Bring the water to boil and the aroma will fill the kitchen. It can simmer away for a number of hours, but you may need to top up the water level every now and again.

For extra special occasions, why not add some cloves, cinnamon sticks and a few pieces of orange and apple peel to the lemon and water while it is simmering in your kitchen. It not only smells delightful, but the vapour spreads around the house and it also humidifies the room.

Spray Freshener

You can make your own spray air-freshener by putting equal amounts of water and lemon juice into a spray bottle. It lasts for ages and is so quick and convenient, plus it smells much more natural than the proprietary air-fresheners. For a more intense freshener you could try adding lemon oil instead of fresh lemon juice.

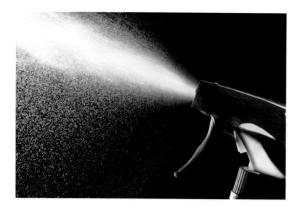

Lemon Oil

Lemon oil can also be good for the mind, levels of concentration and the general feeling of well-being. Try adding a few drops of this essential oil to the water at the top of a ceramic burner as an alternative way to freshen the air in your home. Good for anyone who is having to studying for exams!

Freshen With Light!

Another way of refreshing a room is to put some lemon juice onto a piece of kitchen paper. Then coat your light bulbs with the lemon juice. When the light is turned on the heat from the bulb warms the lemon juice and provides the aroma.

CAUTION: Only apply the lemon juice to light bulbs when they are cold.

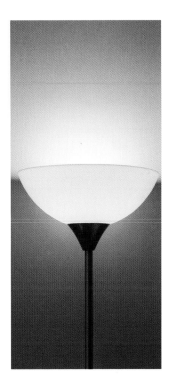

Pop Some in the Wardrobe

To keep clothes and wardrobes smelling delicious, dry out some lemon peel. This may take several days, but once they're really dry put them in a small bowl in the wardrobe, or in the clothes drawer of your dresser.

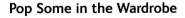

Pop Some in the Vacuum Bag

Freshening as you work must be an added bonus. Sprinkle a few drops of lemon oil onto a piece of kitchen roll, then drop this into the bag of your vacuum cleaner. What a great way to freshen the air all over the house as you clean away the dirt and grime. If you don't have any lemon oil, then a couple of drops of lemon juice will have the same aromatic effect.

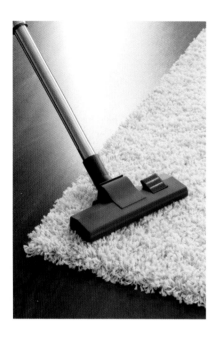

Freshen Carpets and Rugs

While you have the vacuum cleaner out, why not freshen up the carpets and rugs around the home? It does take a little forethought, but it is very effective. Mix together 10 drops of lemon oil, with an equal amount of one of your other favourite essential oils. Add this mixture of sweet-smelling oils to 125 g/4½ oz/1 cup of bicarbonate of soda (baking soda). Bicarbonate of soda (baking soda) is really good at neutralizing smells and the oils provide long-lasting and sweet aromas. Leave the mixture overnight to ensure that the bicarbonate of soda (baking soda) has absorbed all of the oil and then liberally sprinkle it over your carpets and rugs. Let it soak into the tufts of the carpet or rug for a while and then vacuum up the mixture.

Prevent Drains from Smelling

Pour a glass of water containing the juice of a whole lemon down the kitchen sink to keep it fresh-smelling. You can do the same for bath, shower and sink plugholes, because they can also smell, particularly in hot weather. The lemon juice will also disinfect as it travels down the drains.

Eliminate Fireplace Odours

Picture the scene: the wind is howling outside, it is freezing cold and you are sitting beside a warm fire. Absolute joy! But then it starts to belch smoke and the whole room begins to

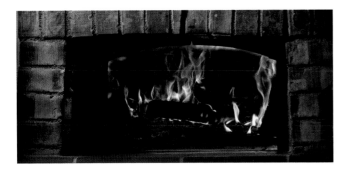

smell like a bonfire! Absolute nightmare! To get rid of that really unpleasant, clogging smell, throw a few pieces of lemon peel into the fire.

You might want to remember to do this as a general rule each time you light the fire, because lemon peel is a good preventative measure against excess smoke. Add it to your firewood when you lay the fire and it will reduce the chance of it happening again.

Get Rid of Mothball Smells

If it's too late and you've already used those smelly mothballs, or in fact have inherited a chest or suitcase from someone who did, it's time for the lemon to the rescue again. Wash the offending areas with lemon juice and water in equal quantities to rid your home of that really unpleasant odour.

Helpful Hints

Remove Scratches on Furniture

You can remove minor scratches on furniture by mixing together equal parts of lemon juice and vegetable oil or olive oil. Rub the mixture onto the affected area quite thoroughly with a soft, dry cloth, then give it a good buff up with another clean cloth. This is also a good recipe for making your own wooden furniture polish. The olive oil leaves a really impressive shine, with the bonus of the clean smell of lemons.

Air Humidifier

If you have an air humidifier you'll know that they are really effective, but they can begin to smell a bit stagnant after a while. Add a few drops of lemon juice to the water in the humidifier to freshen it. The lemony aroma will circulate around the room as the machine does its job.

Holiday Decorations

If you're looking for a project for the December holiday season, you could make your own decorations, using lemons of course. It needs a bit of advance planning, but this project would definitely make your tree unique. In about October put several lemons in a dark cupboard to dry out, making sure you check them from time to time. You could also start to gather pieces of ribbon and pretty, glittering items to stick onto the dried lemons just before the holidays start.

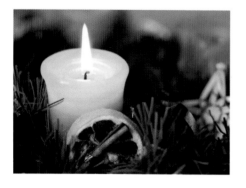

When you're ready to adorn your tree, stick or pin your glittering items into the lemons. Stick a piece of ribbon onto each one to use for hanging and you'll have unique tree decorations!

Easier Holiday Decorations

If you aren't too good at pre-planning or you do not have the time, then you could just make some pomanders to hang. Stick a few cloves into fresh lemons and use ribbon to hang them. You don't have to put them on the tree, they could hang anywhere.

Everyday Decorations

Fresh lemons are such a vibrant colour that they don't always need other items added to make them look attractive. Why not try placing some lemons in an unusually shaped, glass bowl. They look so striking you're sure to get compliments.

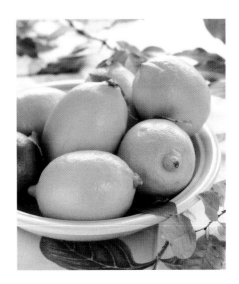

Renew Hardened Paintbrushes

OK, so you had enough of painting the room and you needed a break, but you left the paintbrush overnight and it's now hardened so much that you can't use it. Lemons to the rescue again! Boil some lemon juice in a pan and pop your paintbrush into it for around 15 minutes, simmering away. Turn off the heat and remove the paintbrush, then wash it in hot, soapy water. You'll have bendy bristles again.

Pot Pourri

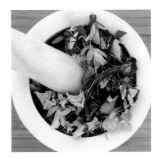

When you buy pot pourri you often find that the smell only lasts for a short while. Why not try adding some dried lemon peel to your favourite dried leaves, flowers or shop-bought pot pourri. To keep it fresh add a few drops of lemon oil onto the peel regularly, or even a few drops of lemon juice will do the job.

Pests & Garden

Ant sprays, mothballs, insecticides, weed killer —

there's an endless list of chemicals we could resort to

if we have an infestation of something we don't want

around the house or garden. But there's really no need

to go to the expense of buying these individual

repellents. Lemons can help eliminate so many

different creepy crawlies. Look what the lemon can rid

you of and then you'll realize why you should always

have a supply of them in your fridge.

Deterring Pests

Natural Insecticide

It may seem strange, but the majority of insects really do not like the smell of lemon. But you do need to be thorough in your application of the lemon juice and peel. Make sure you squeeze liberal amounts of lemon juice on doorsteps and windowsills, as well as any obvious cracks or gaps in the brickwork where you think they could get into the house.

You could also put cut strips of lemon peel around your doorways – why not try the juice and the peel if you really hate creepy crawlies?

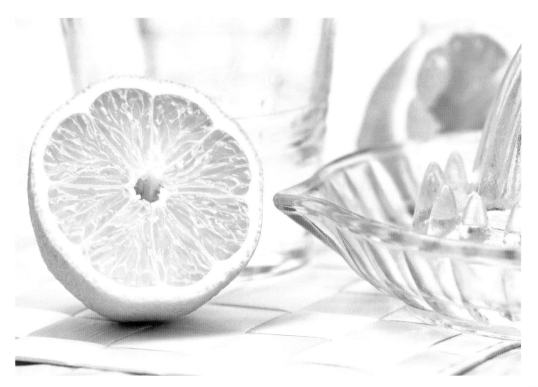

Deter Unwelcome House Guests

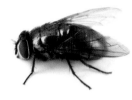

If you've got insects inside the house, and this usually means in the kitchen, perhaps even inside your cupboards, then reach for the lemon again. The limonene in the lemon is toxic to insects, so wipe your surfaces or cupboards with either lemon oil or juice to get rid of them.

Get Rid of Houseflies

We all know how much bacteria the common housefly is capable of spreading around our houses. There is nothing worse than seeing one crawling over kitchen worktops. If you use lemon juice regularly to clean your work surfaces then this will help keep the germ-spreading insects at bay.

Eliminate those Moths!

If you think you might have moths in the wardrobe then don't resort to smelly mothballs. Instead place a small bag of dried lemon peel in the wardrobe. It will help get rid of them.

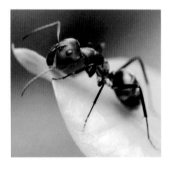

Ant Repellent

Ants don't like lemon either, but the most effective way to rid your house of them is to use a rotten lemon. Place a whole, rotten lemon close to the entrance point they are using to get into your home. You can also squirt your doorways and windowsills with lemon juice, particularly if you can identify where they are entering the house. This organic DIY repellent is also effective against cockroaches and fleas.

Insect-free Paintwork

It has happened to all of us. You're outside giving your home a fresh coat of paint in the summer. You use white gloss paint for the woodwork and you go inside for a coffee only to find on your return that your shiny, white paintwork is covered with tiny bugs and insects. They've stuck to the drying paint. Next time you need to paint outside try rubbing down the door frames or other surfaces you intend to paint with some lemon juice first. It will help keep those little midges away while your paint is drying.

Repel Garden Weeds

Lemon is also good for killing garden weeds. That doesn't mean you are likely to rid your whole garden of them, but lemon juice doused along cracks in pathways and patios will work.

CAUTION: Do not douse any of your garden plants directly with lemon juice as this could harm them.

Squirrel Repellent

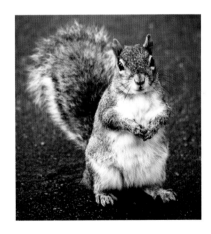

Lemon juice, and some say hot, spicy foods like chilli peppers, can be spread in areas that neighbourhood squirrels frequent regularly. Try placing grated lemon peel around your bird-feeders. They don't like the taste so it will deter them from returning.

If squirrels are causing damage to your flowerbeds, liberally sprinkle grated lemon peel around your plants. It won't hurt the plants but it will stop the squirrels from bothering them.

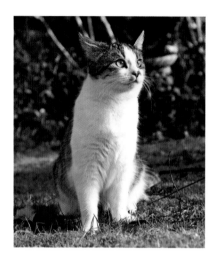

Deter Visiting Cats

Cats do not like the smell of citrus fruit, so using lemon or orange peel in your garden is an effective repellent. Grate and sprinkle liberal amounts of lemon peel where those visiting cats tend to frequent your garden and that should send them back home again.

Train Your Own Cat

If you have a new kitten, or have acquired a stray cat, it is likely that certain parts of your home will be out of bounds for them. Mix some lemon juice and water in a spray bottle and spray it in the areas that you want the cat to avoid. You might have to do this regularly so that they learn.

Gardening

Keep Flowers Fresher

It has been believed for many years that applying proprietary lemonade to pot plants will help ensure they flower for longer. Since then many people also put their cut flowers into lemonade. But you can use fresh lemon juice, too. Try adding 2 tbsp of lemon juice to the water in your vase, together with 1 tbsp of sugar next time you arrange your cut flowers. It does make a difference to the amount of time they stay fresh.

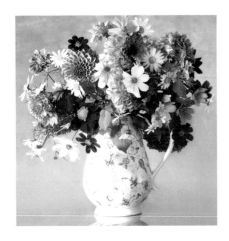

CAUTION: Do not add lemonade or lemon juice to chrysanthemums as this can turn the leaves of the flowers brown.

Improve Soil Quality

There are lots of bags of compost available in garden centres, but many people choose to make their own. If you make your own organic compost you will realize it is much better for your garden soil than those that contain chemicals. The secret to good-quality soil is good-quality compost. Adding citrus fruit to the compost can help improve soil quality enormously because it enriches the soil with nutrients. The lemon, orange or grapefruit will help to regulate the flow of water and oxygen to the roots of the plants. This will obviously give you a healthier plant, which will also be less prone to pests and diseases.

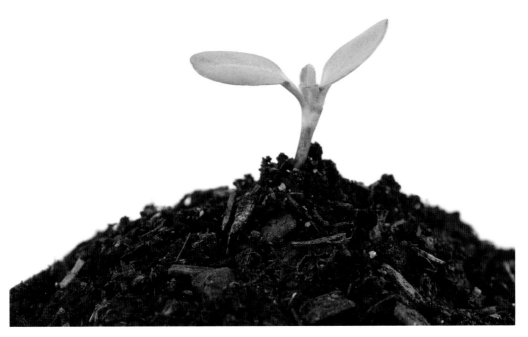

Pet Care

Having healthy and well-behaved pets is probably as important to most pet owners as their own health. We are a nation of animal lovers, after all! Of course you can buy many pet-care products that probably do work, but they can be expensive and you don't always know what ingredients they contain. The natural and easily available lemon gives you lots of options for protecting your pet's health, and can be useful in different methods of training.

Cats & Dogs

Lemon Spray for Dogs

Lemon is very effective for conditioning a dog's coat and keeping your pet flea free. Add slices of lemon to ½ litre/1 pint/2 cups of boiling water and leave the mixture to cool by letting it stand overnight. Strain the mixture and then pour it into a spray bottle. You can spray your animal liberally with this mixture without it having any harmful effects. The limonene in the lemon conditions the dog's coat and it is also an effective repellent for flies and other flying insects. This spray is also very effective for keeping away animal fleas. These unwanted little creatures have a waxy coating. When the liquid is sprayed onto the animal's fur it disables the flea from feeding.

CAUTION: Avoid spraying the lemon juice mixture near to the dog's eyes.

Cat-box Cleaner

Cat litter boxes are a brilliant idea, but they can get a bit overpowering if they're not cleaned regularly and properly. The problem is they tend to get a layer of scale in the base. Try using a mixture of white vinegar, water and freshly squeezed lemon juice in the cat box next time you clean it. Use 3 parts water to 1 part white vinegar and the juice of 2 lemons. Transfer this mixture to a spray bottle and after you've emptied and washed the box with

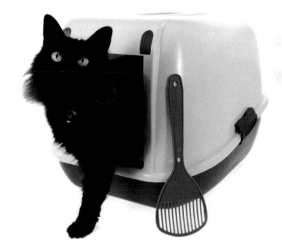

warm, soapy water, spray the base of it with the mixture. Then scrub the base with a stiff brush, wash again and rinse the box thoroughly. The sediment will come off easily and the box will stay fresher for longer.

CAUTION: Do make sure you clean off the lemon thoroughly, as cats are not keen on the smell of lemon and you don't want to deter them from using the box.

Protect Dog's Ears from Damage Whilst Swimming

If your dog is a keen swimmer, the chances are that water in the ears might be or has been a problem. You can protect your pet's ears by using a lemon flush. Mix together the juice of half a lemon with some warm water. You will need to use an ear dropper, or even a syringe, to administer the mixture. Gently squeeze some of the liquid into each of your pet's ears and, again gently, massage the outside of the ear to rub it in. Your pet will probably have a good shake at this stage, at which point you can blot away the excess moisture with cotton wool or a cotton bud.

CAUTION: Do not place the syringe or ear dropper right inside your pet's ear canal as the squirting noise might frighten it and the ear canal is very delicate.

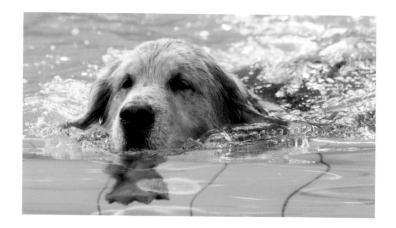

Train Your Dog to Stop Barking

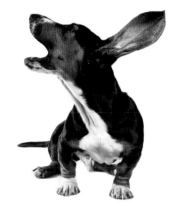

You can buy anti-barking collars that contain citronella. These squirt into the dog's face every time it barks to deter it from excessive barking. However it is much cheaper and probably just as effective to make your own version using a water pistol or spray bottle and some lemon juice. Fill the water pistol or spray bottle with water and add a few drops of lemon juice. The spray isn't meant to be a punishment but is meant to startle the dog into silence by interrupting the barking. Every time the dog barks you spray the lemon mixture into his or her mouth and praise when the barking stops. If the barking begins again, repeat the process.

CAUTION: Do not spray the lemon juice and water mixture directly into the dog's face and be careful to avoid the eyes.

Stop Puppies from Biting Your Hands

Because dogs do not like the taste of lemon, you could try rubbing lemon juice into your hands if you have one that likes to gnaw your fingers. It might take two or three goes before your puppy realizes, but it will stop them biting your hands eventually.

Pet Potty Training

If your puppy tends to use one particular area of the house as his or her private toilet, then you can use lemon juice to deter them from doing so. The trouble is if they do it in the same place time and time again then it can become the norm. Spray the area with neat lemon juice, which won't hurt your floor or carpet. The smell will eliminate the odour in your home and will also deter the animal from returning to its own scent.

Health & Personal Care

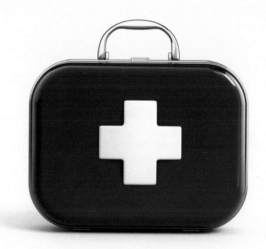

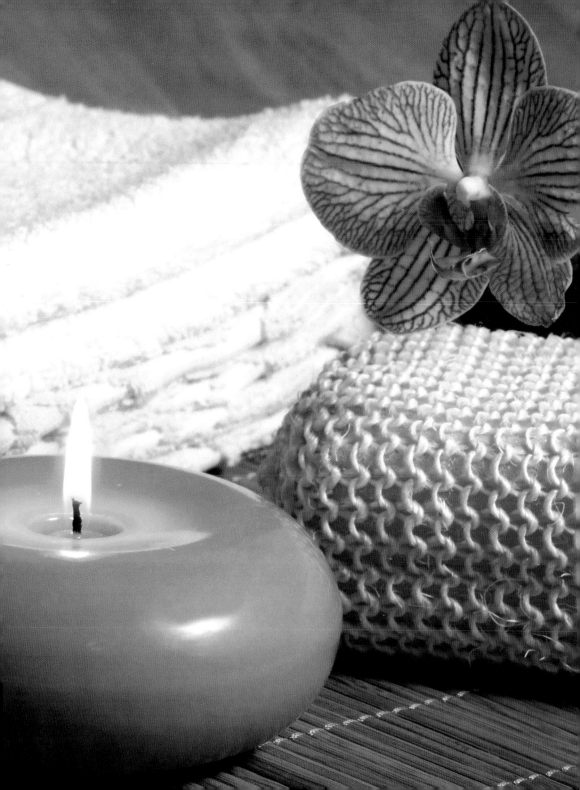

Beauty Tips

All parts of a lemon contain something that we can use to make ourselves look and feel beautiful. We can use lemon on our hair, our skin and our nails. And not just for one thing – lemon juice is a truly diverse organic beauty aid. It can cleanse, moisturize, help maintain the pH balance in skin and soften it. But perhaps more importantly it can help us maintain a healthy body. What more could you expect from a piece of fruit?

Skin

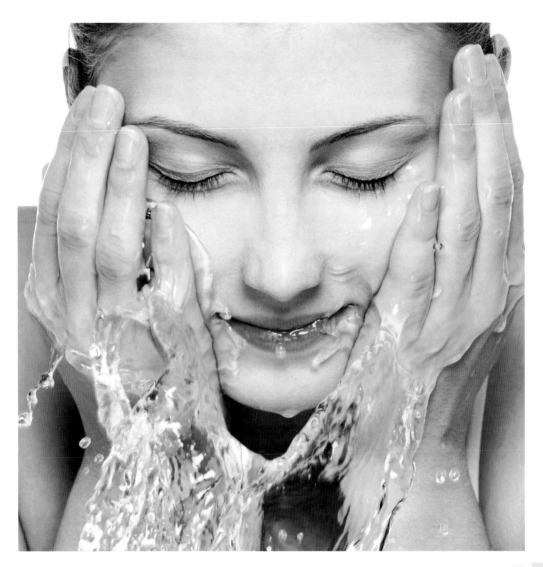

Cleansing

Lemons have a strong reputation for being particularly good at cleansing and they also have clarifying properties. Lemon juice can help remove dead skin cells and stimulate collagen production. You could use this lemon cleansing treatment every day to remove the dirt and grime that has built up on your face. Squeeze the juice from half a lemon into a bowl and apply to your face with your fingertips. Gently massage the lemon juice into your pores and then rinse your face.

CAUTION: Do not cleanse the area around the eyes with lemon juice, as this could cause stinging.

Deep Cleansing

Lemons are particularly useful for combatting greasy skin as they are great for unclogging pores. The lemon oil helps to balance overactive sebaceous glands, which are often what

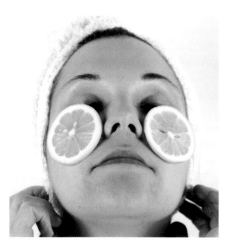

cause greasy skin, blocked pores and skin blemishes. One good method of deep cleansing to make sure those pores are cleaned thoroughly is to steam the face. Fill a bowl with boiling water and add the peel of half a lemon. With your face over the bowl and a tea towel over your head, let the lemony steam penetrate the pores. You'll be amazed at how refreshing this feels, too!

Toning

Once you've cleansed your face you'll want to tone it to close those pores up again. Use two

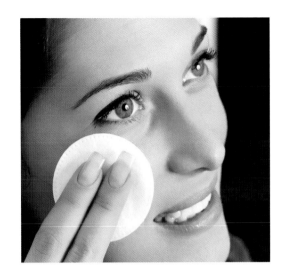

parts ice-cold water to one part lemon juice to tone after cleansing. Apply the cold toner to clean skin and allow it to dry naturally. Can you imagine how good this toner makes you feel on a really hot day? You can store this cold, lemony toner in the refrigerator for several days.

CAUTION: Do not be tempted to go into the sunshine after using lemon on the face because the lemon juice can react to the sun's UV rays and burn or blemish the skin.

Toning Oily Skin

For oily skin, mix 2 tbsp of lemon juice, 2 tbsp of vodka, 1 tbsp of distilled water and 1 tsp of witch hazel. Use a cotton wool pad to apply this toner to your skin and then rinse your face with water. This toner will also keep for around a week if stored in the refrigerator.

Moisturizing

Lemon juice moisturizes as well as cleanses and tones. It is the lemon acids that are good at moisturizing because they help the skin to prevent water loss. Lemon can help soften and smooth even the driest skin. Smooth the lemon juice over the skin, either with your fingertips or cotton wool, and let it dry before rinsing off. If you don't have time to squeeze the lemon, just chop it in half and apply the lemon directly to your face, squeezing a little to release the juice.

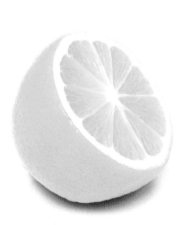
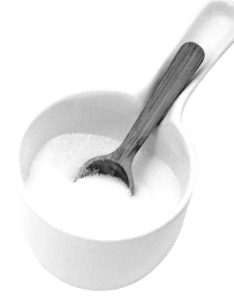

Face Exfoliator

To get rid of dead facial skin cells, cut a lemon in half and dip it into ordinary white sugar. Using this as your exfoliator, gently rub your face to remove the build up of dead skin. If you do this regularly you'll notice the difference. The lemon juice is really good at loosening dead skin cells and the sugar acts as a mild abrasive. Do it at bedtime though, so you don't risk being in the sunlight immediately afterwards.

CAUTION: If you have any skin sensitivity, try a test patch for any of these lemon treatments first, as they are quite acidic.

Freckle Lightener

There are two ways of using lemon juice to lighten freckles. You can use it to exfoliate dead skin, which will diminish the appearance of the freckles. Gently rub a cut lemon and half a teaspoon of sugar granules over the skin. Repeat this once a week, until the freckles begin to fade.

Alternatively, apply a slice of lemon to the freckled area of the skin and leave it to do its job for about 10 minutes. Repeat this weekly and you are sure to see the freckles begin to lighten.

CAUTION: Using neat lemon juice on the skin can dry it out, so make sure you moisturize after treating your freckles.

Wrinkle Reducers

Lemons can be used in a number of different ways to help improve the appearance of wrinkles. One of the simplest methods is to stir a teaspoon of sugar into 2 tbsp of lemon juice. Massage this solution into your skin using your fingertips. Leave the mix on your face for 10 minutes before rinsing off with water. This treatment will exfoliate the skin, but the Vitamin C in the lemon will also promote the production of collagen. Acids in the sugar will help repair skin damage and also remove dead skin.

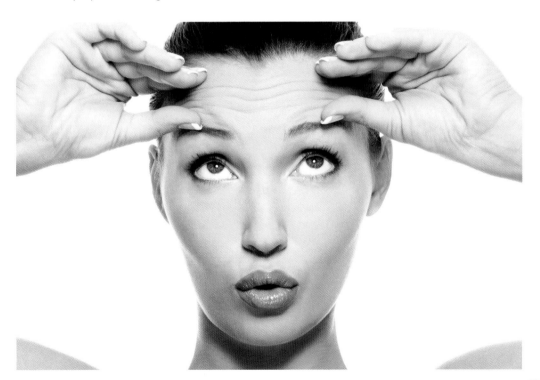

Another home-made remedy for wrinkles and fine lines on the face is to mix together 1 tsp of tomato juice, ½ tsp of lemon juice and a pinch of turmeric. Form this into a paste with gram or chickpea flour. Apply the paste to the wrinkled area, and leave for 15 to 20 minutes before washing off.

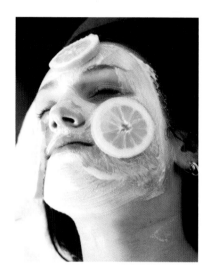

Using lemon juice as an essential ingredient for a facial mask also helps reduce wrinkles. Add 1 tbsp of lemon juice to a well-beaten egg white and 1 tsp of egg yolk. Add a drop of Vitamin E oil into this mix and form a paste. Apply the paste to the skin and leave for 30 minutes before washing off. Moisturize your face after you have used this wrinkle treatment.

One further anti-wrinkle treatment requires a little more time and preparation. You will need several lemons, two cucumbers, whipped cream, olive oil, honey and corn starch (corn flour). Slice the unpeeled cucumbers and put them into a blender, together with the whipped cream, and blitz until you have a paste. Add a drop or two of olive oil and honey and continue blitzing before adding just a pinch of corn starch (corn flour). Now put the mixture into the refrigerator and let it chill for at least 30 minutes. When you are ready for this luxurious anti-wrinkle treatment, cut the lemons in half and begin rubbing them generously but lightly over your neck and face. Don't dry the skin and apply the paste mixture straightaway. Leave the mix to do its job for at least an hour before rinsing it off.

Pimple and Blackhead Remover

Lemon juice is an excellent astringent and it can help remove dirt that can clog your pores. We all know that clogged pores can cause blackheads and pimples, but there are natural ways that lemons can help.

Squeeze the juice of half a lemon into a small bowl, then dip a cotton wool ball into the juice and dab it onto your face, taking care to avoid your eyes. You can either leave it on for around 10 minutes before washing it off, or you can do this just before you go to bed at night. Leave the lemon juice to soak in overnight before rinsing off in the morning. The citric acid in the lemon juice will naturally dissolve the oils that conspire to create blackheads. See below for a useful regular facial mask to treat blackheads.

Cleansing Facial Masks

Here are two simple recipes to create easy-to-use cleansing masks with lemon as one of the main ingredients.

As a regular treatment for blackheads mix 2 tbsp of oatmeal with 4 tbsp of plain yoghurt, and 1 tbsp of lemon juice. Mix the ingredients into a paste and apply to the skin. Leave this cleansing facial mask on for at least five minutes, then rinse off with cold water. Either pat the face dry or leave it to air dry naturally.

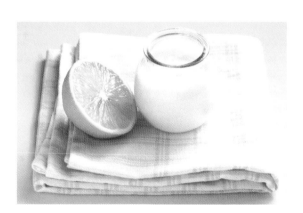
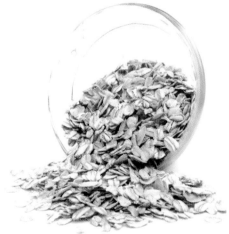

For deep cleansing, mix 4 tbsp of plain yoghurt with 2 tbsp of grated lemon peel. Massage this mask into your skin and leave on the face for up to five minutes, then rinse off with warm water. During this deep cleanse the lemon peel dissolves the dirt and oil and the yoghurt exfoliates your skin.

Dark Spots Lightener

Lemon juice is one of the most natural and potent skin-bleaching products available. Squeeze a lemon into a small container or spray bottle. Dilute the lemon juice with an equal amount of water. Optionally you can add a drop of honey or aloe vera oil, as these are both useful moisturizers. Apply the lemon mixture to a test area first, such as the neck, and then rinse it off. If the test patch proves to be problem free then apply the mixture to the darker spots you wish to lighten. Leave the mixture on for a minute or two before rinsing off with water. Make sure you then moisturize your skin well. You can repeat this treatment weekly.

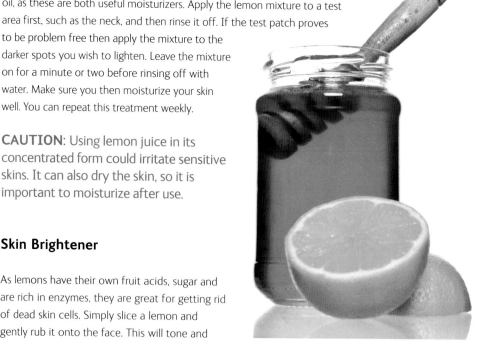

CAUTION: Using lemon juice in its concentrated form could irritate sensitive skins. It can also dry the skin, so it is important to moisturize after use.

Skin Brightener

As lemons have their own fruit acids, sugar and are rich in enzymes, they are great for getting rid of dead skin cells. Simply slice a lemon and gently rub it onto the face. This will tone and refresh the skin. Wash off the lemon juice after this treatment.

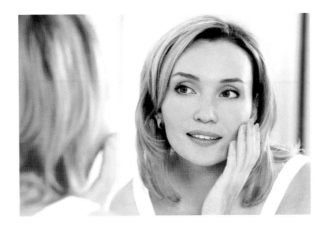

Shiny Face Reducer

Brush your face with lemon juice using a clean makeup brush. Leave the juice on your skin for five minutes before rinsing off. The lemon juice will help deal with the over production of oil in the skin. As an alternative, use 120 ml/4 fl oz/½ cup of water mixed with 10 drops of lemon juice. Using a cotton wool ball, dab the mixture all over the face.

CAUTION: If you are using neat lemon juice do this last thing at night, as the lemon juice may cause a temporary redness of the skin.

Age-spot Reducer

If you have dark spots on the skin, which can be caused by over-exposure to the sun ('age spots' or 'liver spots'), try mixing 1 tbsp of yoghurt with a drop or two of lemon juice. Apply the mixture directly to the age spot and leave for 10 minutes before rinsing off.

An alternative treatment is to simply dab fresh lemon juice directly onto the age spots twice a day. Leave the juice on the skin for as long as you like and you should notice improvements after around two months of daily treatment.

CAUTION: If the lemon juice stings the skin you should rinse it off immediately and remember not to go straight into the sunlight.

Body Exfoliator

This may sound more like a torture treatment than a beauty aid, but it is great for getting rid of those dead cells. Prepare in advance a mixture of 225 g/8 oz/¾ cup of sea salt with ½ tbsp of lemon oil and put it beside the bath. Draw yourself a warm bath. Rub your damp skin with the lemon-scented salt. This will deal with dead skin cells and give your skin a smooth and healthy glow.

You could try adding coconut oil or almond oil in addition to the lemon oil to give you a really sumptuous-smelling body scrub for the bath.

Body Massage

In addition to all the other wonderful things we've learned about, lemons are also believed to help the skin's elasticity and discourage cellulite. Try mixing equal amounts of honey,

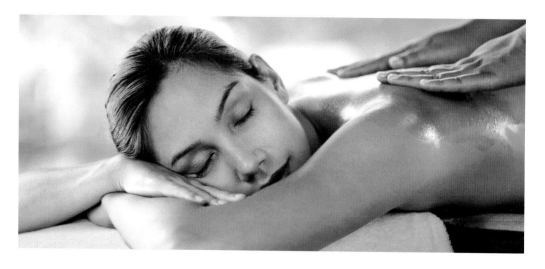

vegetable oil and lemon juice together. Use this as your massage oil and pay particular attention to those areas of the body that are particularly dry. Leave the mixture on your body for about 10 minutes before rinsing it off in the shower or a warm bath.

Dark Underarms and Elbows

We've already seen how lemon juice can help reduce dark patches on the skin (see page 86). If you have discoloured elbows or dark patches of skin under the armpit then lemons can also help.

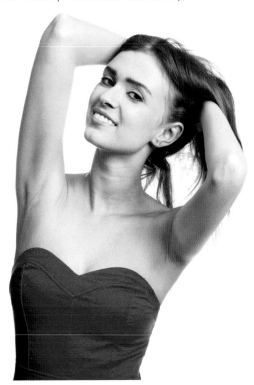

For elbows, cut a lemon in half and rest your elbows in each half for 10 minutes. Rinse off with warm water.

For discoloured armpits cut a thick slice of lemon and clamp your arm against your body, trapping the lemon slice. Leave for 10 minutes. Rinse off with warm water. You can repeat both of these treatments regularly until the darker skin gradually lightens.

Short-term Deodorant

In an emergency, lemons can be used as a short-term deodorizer. Either dab a little lemon extract to freshen up your armpits, or rub a wedge of lemon onto the skin of the armpit. It will only last for a few hours, but it is effective.

Hair & Nails

Help With Dandruff

There are two ways that lemons can rid you of an itching scalp and embarrassing dandruff flakes on the shoulders.

Try adding 2 tbsp of lemon juice to 120 ml/4 fl oz/½ cup of olive oil. Gently rub the mixture onto your scalp and leave it for about 15 minutes before rinsing off. Then you can shampoo and condition your hair as normal.

Alternatively, mix a few drops of lemon juice into an egg white. Apply the mixture to your scalp and rub it in. Leave the mix on your scalp for around an hour before shampooing your hair with lukewarm water and then rinsing. You can repeat this procedure four or five times a month to help eliminate dandruff.

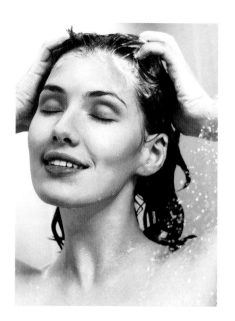

Reduce Hair Loss

Hair loss can be tackled by using a combination of lemon juice and coconut milk. Mix the juice of one lemon to 4 tbsp of coconut milk. Apply the mixture to the scalp at least once a week. Rinse your hair with warm water to remove the mixture and then shampoo and condition as normal.

Sun-Kissed Hair

Lemons are natural bleaching agents. All you need to do is to squeeze the juice of half to a whole lemon straight onto your hair. Sit out in the sun for at least 30 minutes and then shampoo and condition your hair as normal. Alternatively, mix 4 tbsp of lemon juice with 175 ml/6 fl oz/¾ cup of water, then rinse your clean, wet hair with the mixture. Sit out in the sun until your hair dries.

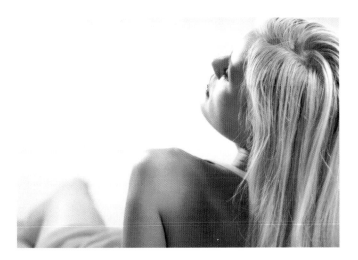

If you are light haired, blonde highlights will begin to appear. If you are darker haired, then you will see red tones begin to appear in the hair.

Hair Shampoo

You can make your own home-made shampoo with lemon juice as the vital ingredient. Mix a whole egg with 1 tsp of olive oil, 1 tsp of lemon juice, 120 ml/4 fl oz/½ cup of warm water and a few small pieces of your favourite soap, or a squirt of liquid soap. If you are using pieces of soap, soak them in the warm water until they are soft before adding the remaining ingredients.

Your home-made shampoo will last for up to three days, and even longer if it is kept in the refrigerator.

Hair Conditioner

There are at least a couple of ways of making your own hair conditioner using lemons. If you have dull or damaged hair, mix together 3 tbsp of lemon juice, 120 ml/4 fl oz/½ cup of honey and 200 ml/7 fl oz/¾ cup of olive oil. Shampoo your hair as normal and then towel dry. Apply the mixture to your hair and comb it through. Cover your hair with a plastic cap and leave for 30 minutes. Then shampoo and rinse your hair as normal.

For a more general hair conditioner, use one egg, the juice of half a lemon, 1 tbsp of olive oil and 3 tbsp of henna powder. Beat the egg until it is frothy, then slowly add the henna powder and the lemon juice. You may need to add a few drops of water at this stage if the mixture feels too stiff. Allow the mixture to set for an hour before using it. Apply to your hair and scalp, and leave it on for an hour before rinsing and shampooing.

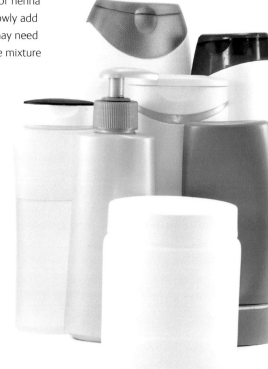

Shiny Hair

This treatment is particularly effective if you have greasy hair. After you have shampooed, rinse with a little water and the juice of half a lemon. The lemon's natural acidity will counteract the alkaline traces of the shampoo. It will also dissolve any residual soap and help to create fatty acids that will give your hair a natural shine.

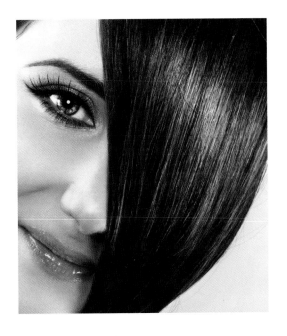

Treating Damaged or Coloured Hair

Bleaches and colouring agents can often damage your hair. Rinsing with water and the juice of half a lemon encourages natural proteins, which can counteract hair damage.

Scalp Treatment

This is an effective hair and scalp treatment for all hair types. Mix an egg with 2 tbsp of honey, 2 tbsp of olive oil, 1 tbsp of lemon juice and a drop of two or your favourite essential oil. Mix everything together in a bowl and apply the mix over the hair and scalp. Leave for at least 20 minutes (but no longer than 40 minutes), then shampoo with lukewarm water. Finally give your hair and scalp a cold-water rinse. You can substitute the olive oil for sesame, coconut or almond oil if you wish.

Natural Hairspray

A great lemony hairspray, which works for all types of hair, is very simple to make. Slice four lemons and put them into a saucepan with 900 ml/1^1/$_2$ pints/3¾ cups of water. Simmer the mixture for 15 minutes, or until around half the water has evaporated. Then strain the liquid into a spray bottle and add a few drops of your favourite essential oil. Keep the spray bottle in the refrigerator and it should last for at least a week.

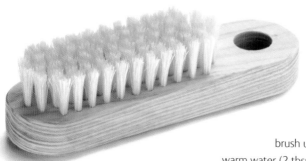

Shiny Nails

To get lovely shiny nails, soak your fingernails (or toenails) in lemon juice for 10 minutes, and brush them with a toothbrush or a small nail brush using a mixture of white wine vinegar and warm water (2 tbsp each), mixed with the juice of half a lemon. It will help your nails stay bright, strong and shiny. This is also a good way of removing the yellow colour that develops with the regular use of nail polish.

Smoking and using nail polish can lead to discoloured nails. Simply cut a fresh lemon and squeeze the juice into a shallow bowl. Soak your nails and fingertips in the lemon juice for several minutes. Repeat this over a number of days to rid your nails of any yellowing. After each treatment wash and rinse your hands and apply a moisturizer.

Strong Nails

To soften your cuticles and strengthen your nails at the same time add 3 tbsp of freshly squeezed lemon juice to a little liquid soap. Add a few drops of warm water and soak your nails in this mixture for five minutes. This will leave your fingers feeling soft and your nails strong and healthy looking.

If you have brittle fingernails, try rubbing sliced lemon every day on them. This will help your nails become much stronger and sturdier.

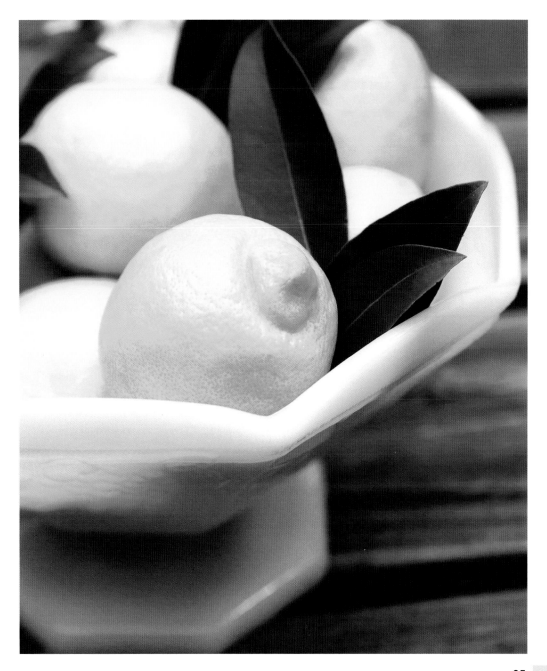

Natural Remedies

We all know the old wives' tale, 'an apple a day keeps the doctor away'. But it is not just apples that are good for us. Eating a raw lemon is not particularly recommended, but lemons can be used for a whole range of health conditions. Lemons are anti-fungal, anti-viral, antioxidant, anti-cancer, anti-inflammatory and antihistamine. They are also diuretics, detoxifiers and tonics. Look at the huge range of natural lemon remedies to see just how versatile this fruit can be. We have listed them in alphabetical order.

Head & Face

Sore and Puffy Eyes

Of course it is never advisable to put neat lemon juice into the eyes, but adding a drop or two of lemon juice to a cup of warm water will do you no harm. Simply use the solution as you would a normal eye wash to soothe sore eyes.

If your eyes are a bit puffy, maybe from hay fever or a particularly late night, try squeezing the juice of a lemon into a small bowl. Add two slices of cucumber to the lemon juice and let the slices sit in the juice for a minute or two. Place one of the cucumber slices over each eye and relax. This will not only get rid of puffy eyes, but will also help to reduce dark circles underneath the eyes.

Chapped Lips

Chapped lips can sting and make you feel very miserable in the winter months. Place a small amount of Vaseline or glycerine onto a saucer and mix in the juice of half a lemon. Apply your home-made lip balm to your lips to heal and soothe.

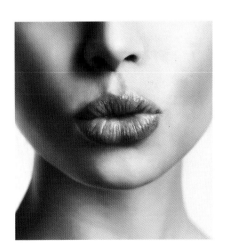

Cold Sores

Lemons have been used to deal with cold sores for generations. Simply cut a slice of lemon and place it directly onto the affected spot. It will sting, but try to keep it there for as long as you can bear it. Change the slice and reapply.

To help avoid cold sores from developing, try squeezing four lemons into a glass of water for a daily drink. This will give your body an extra boost that will both prevent and treat cold sores.

CAUTION: Only apply the lemon slice treatment at the beginning of a cold sore outbreak. Do not use on open sores or broken skin.

Gum Disease and Other Mouth Problems

You will need to brace yourself for this because it involves chewing the peel of a lemon! The natural healing properties of lemons will act on your gums and strengthen them, as well as killing off and inhibiting mouth bacteria, which can cause gum disease.

Fresh lemon juice can also be applied if you have a toothache. The sharp, tangy liquid will help reduce the pain.

If you massage lemon juice onto bleeding gums it will help stop the bleeding.

Earache

For an effective remedy for earache, squeeze a little lemon juice and add to a similar amount of mustard oil. Heat the two fluids together until you have an oily residue. When you have earache put a couple of drops into the ear and this will help ease the pain.

Nose Bleeds

The lemon's peel, pith and core can help strengthen blood vessels and lemon juice has strong astringent properties. If you have a nose bleed, soak a cotton wool ball in lemon juice and put the ball into the affected nostril. Leave the cotton wool ball in your nostril for at least 10 minutes. The lemon juice will help to seal the broken blood vessels by tightening up the membranes in your nose.

Head Lice

The horror of head lice can be averted by simply adding two drops of lemon oil into your shampoo. Then add another two drops into your hair conditioner. The presence of the acidic lemon will help to deter the outbreak of an infestation of head lice or make life uncomfortable for them if they have already arrived.

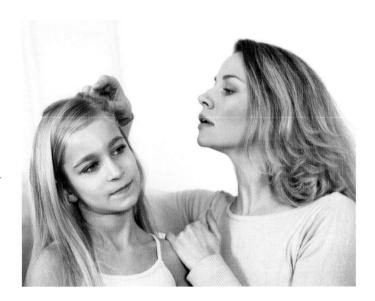

Hands & Feet

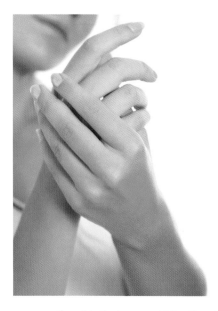

Dry Hands

If you have dry hands, simply squeeze the juice of a lemon into a bowl of warm water. Dunk your hands into the soothing mixture. Keep your hands immersed for two or three minutes, then dry them off and pour a little olive oil into the palm of your hand. Gently rub in the olive oil, massaging it into your hands.

Fingertip Splits

Fingertip splits can really hurt. Lemon oil can not only speed their healing, but will also soften the skin and soothe. All you need to do is to bury your finger tip in a piece of lemon peel. This will release the oil in the lemon, which will soak into the split skin wound. Repeat the process two or three times a day until the split is healed.

Chilblains

Chilblains are caused by fluid leaking out of tiny blood vessels into your skin. Lemons can help reduce the swelling and the itchy sensation. All you need to do is make sure that you include lemon juice and zest in your everyday diet.

Aching Feet

Make yourself a wonderful foot soak
by squeezing the juice of a lemon into
a bowl of warm water. After soaking
the feet, massage them with olive oil.
This also works if your hands are
extremely dry.

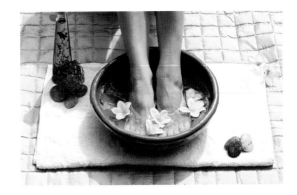

Soothe Sore Feet

After an exhausting days' shopping, your feet might be grateful for the soothing and healing
properties of a lemon. If your feet are sore, rub a sliced lemon over the burning part of the
foot to relieve the pain and eliminate any toxins.

You can also soak your feet in warm water to which the juice of a whole lemon has been added.
This will help to cool the feet and promote a good nights' sleep by relaxing the throbbing.

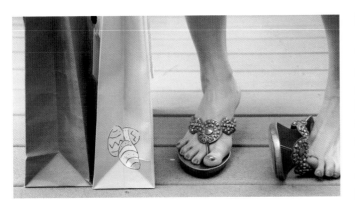

Swollen Ankles

There can be many
reasons why your ankles
might swell; there could
be an underlying problem
that results in fluid
retention, so of course it
is always best to consult
your doctor if this is a
persistent problem.

However, lemons can help strengthen the walls of veins and they are also a diuretic, which encourages the production of urine. This will help reduce fluid retention. To help prevent swollen ankles, include lemons, particularly the juice and zest, in your daily diet.

Athlete's Foot

Lemon juice can help in dealing with this irritating fungal infection. Soak a cotton wool ball in lemon juice and apply directly to the infected area, or squeeze the juice of a lemon into a bowl of warm water or foot bath and bathe your feet in it for ten minutes.

Corns

Corns can be extremely painful and, if ignored, they could cause all sorts of foot problems. Lemons are good for dealing with corns and calluses. You can either apply neat lemon juice directly three times a day, or you can use lemon oil as an accelerating process.

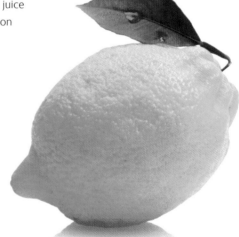

The overnight alternative is to place either a slice of lemon or the peel of a lemon onto the corn and stick it in place with a plaster.

CAUTION: When applying lemon oil always make sure that the undiluted oil is only applied to the corn or callus, as it could damage normal skin.

Skin

Acne

The over-production of sebum can encourage infection and cause acne. Lemon juice helps to kill the bacteria and it also reduces inflammation and emulsifies the oils in the skin. Simply squeeze the juice of a lemon into a small bowl and soak it up with a cotton wool ball. Apply the juice to the affected areas two or three times a day.

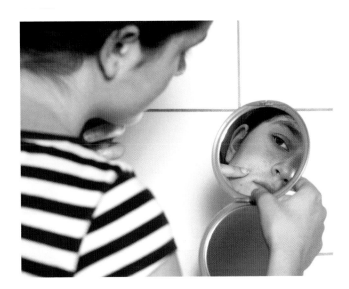

Psoriasis

The citric acid in lemon juice should help ease flaky and dry skin and also help deal with the underlying inflammation caused by psoriasis. As an anti-inflammatory, applying neat lemon juice to psoriasis patches several times a day and then exposing those patches to direct sunlight for a few minutes will help.

This is a home-cure version of a similar treatment used by dermatologists. Those with psoriasis should certainly incorporate lemons into their regular daily diet, too.

Eczema

Eczema is a very irritating skin infection. You can create a lemon wrap to relieve your skin from this itching by either squeezing the juice of a whole lemon or four drops of lemon oil into 250 ml/8 fl oz/1 cup of warm water and 1 tbsp of honey. Soak a

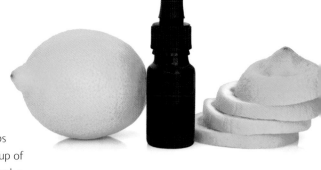

clean cloth in the liquid and squeeze out the excess. Place the cloth over the affected area and leave it there for 15 minutes.

You can repeat this process two or three times a day. This brilliant mixture will not only ease the infection but it will stop you from wanting to scratch. The lemon will heal and the honey acts as an anti-inflammatory, too. Another way to relieve itchy skin is to squeeze the juice of two lemons into a warm bath and have a soak.

CAUTION: Eczema can cause broken skin often due to scratching, which may be aggravated by lemon juice. Also, people with sensitive skin, who are prone to conditions such as eczema and psoriasis, are often allergic or intolerant to citrus fruits. Anyone with a strong and persistent problem with eczema and psoriasis should consult their dermatologist or doctor before using any of these lemon-based treatments.

Anti-Ageing

Lemons are a wonderful source of Vitamin C. This vitamin encourages the body to make collagen, which is used to build joints, bones, ligaments and blood vessels. By ensuring that lemons are part of your daily diet your body will be more able to repair muscles and keep them healthy, as well as giving your skin every chance to stay fresh and youthful.

Cellulite

Lemon juice is ideal for a wide range of skin problems. Cellulite is a dimpling of the skin where there is excess tissue fluid. Massage lemon oil onto the affected area. As lemons are rich in Vitamin C and also act as a diuretic, you can either make sure that you include lemon juice and zest in your daily diet, or add two drops of lemon oil to your bath water and rub the dimpled skin area with a loofah. Using lemon juice in this way should reduce excess tissue fluid and therefore cellulite marks.

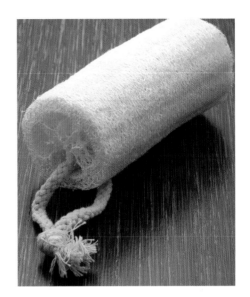

Broken Veins

Lemon juice or lemon oil is very effective for treating circulatory problems, such as broken capillaries, or spider veins. Lemons contain Vitamin P in the peel and the juice, so lemons are great for keeping your capillaries strong and strengthening the arterial system. For spider veins add two or three drops of lemon oil to jojoba or almond oil and massage into the affected area.

Varicose Veins

The natural astringent and anti-inflammatory qualities of the lemon will strengthen the walls of veins. To help reduce the appearance of varicose veins, mix two drops of lemon oil with three drops of cypress oil and two drops of lavender oil, along with 2 tbsp of almond oil. Massage the mixture directly onto the area affected by the varicose veins. Repeat the treatment once a day until you begin to see results.

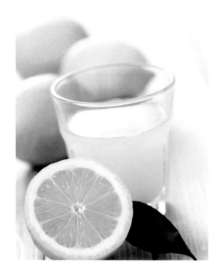

Wart Removal

If you are prone to warts, a preventative measure is to drink the juice of a whole lemon each day. You can, of course, water this down, and perhaps add a dash of sugar to make it more palatable.

For generations people have thought that rubbing a potato onto a wart and then burying the potato is a sure-fire wart cure. What certainly does work is rubbing lemon juice directly onto the wart and covering it with a plaster. Repeat the procedure every day for at least two weeks. Slowly but surely the lemon juice will dissolve the wart.

Bruises

Lemon peel and lemon juice can actually limit bruising and also speed the recovery from a bruise. Either rub lemon peel onto the affected area, or include the juice of a lemon and its zest in your regular diet.

Burn Marks

Burns are painful and can cause swelling, redness or even blisters. If you burn your hand on the oven, or touch the iron, turn to lemon juice for the solution. All you will need is lemon juice, tomato extract and almond oil.

Rinse the burn under cool, running water and cover the mark with a dampened cloth. Then dampen the cloth with lemon juice and apply it to the burn. This will help to cleanse the skin and lighten the burn mark. Repeat this treatment to thoroughly cleanse the area before rubbing tomato extract onto the burn mark. The tomato will naturally bleach the area. To complete the recovery process, apply some almond oil to soften the skin, improve the skin colour and remove what is left of the burn mark. This treatment should not only help to heal the burn, but also accelerate the skin lightening process. You can use the pulp of a tomato instead of tomato extract and coconut oil instead of almond oil if you prefer.

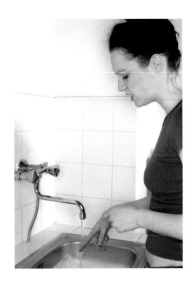

Cuts and Grazes

Lemons are great antiseptics. The juice alone will deal with most minor cuts and grazes. They are also excellent for mouth ulcers. If you have a larger cut, rub either lemon peel or juice into the affected area. This will sting, but on the upside it will kill any infection and help soothe the inflammation.

Insect Bites

Lemon juice will not only reduce the itching caused by insect bites, but it will also bring down any swelling. If you have been bitten by a cloud of mosquitoes, squeeze the juice of two lemons into a warm bath and bathe in it to reduce the itching and subsequent swelling.

For other stings and bites, such as from a wasp, apply neat lemon juice with a cotton wool pad directly onto the bite site. Repeat this as often as necessary to bring down the inflammation and swelling.

Lemon juice mixed with eucalyptus oil is also believed to be a great mosquito repellent.

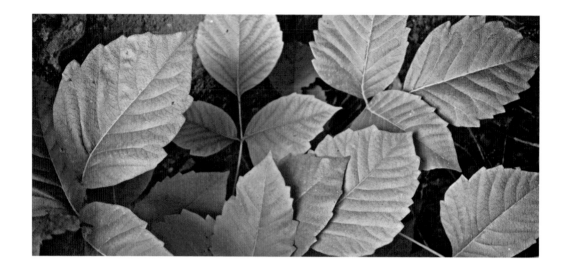

Poison Ivy

Poison ivy can give you a dreadful rash. The traditional treatment is to use camomile lotion, but lemons are quicker, easier to obtain and more effective.

Squeeze the juice of a lemon into a bowl. Dunk a cotton wool pad into the juice and apply it directly to the rash area to reduce the inflammation and soothe the itching sensation.

Scars

Lemon and cucumber juice can be combined to help remove scarring, or at least to reduce the impact of a visible scar.

Squeeze the juice of a lemon into a bowl and then add an equal amount of cucumber juice (to obtain the cucumber juice, grate the cucumber and then squeeze the juice from the pulp

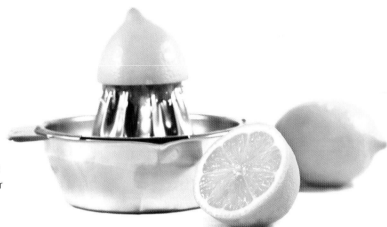

by wringing it in a dish towel) into the same bowl and mix. Gently dab the mixture onto the scarred tissue. Leave it to dry for up to 10 minutes, then wash off with water and pat dry. Repeat the treatment on a daily basis until the scar begins to fade.

CAUTION: Do not apply to freshly scarred areas or those that still have stitches in them.

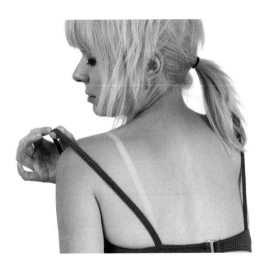

Sunburn Relief

As lemon juice is such an efficient astringent, its healing properties will help calm irritated, sunburned skin. Squeeze the juice of a lemon into a bowl and add three times the amount of water. Apply this gently and directly onto the sunburned skin using a cotton wool pad.

If you have badly burned your skin, then add three drops of lemon oil to 2 tbsp of almond oil and apply this to the sunburned area.

Internal Health

CAUTION: It is important to remember that all uses of lemons on the body, especially internally and for serious conditions, should be practised with caution and do not replace the advice of a doctor.

Anaemia

If you are iron deficient then you may have a low level of stomach acid. The acidity in a lemon can help by lowering the pH level in your stomach. The pectin in a lemon is broken down by bacteria in the stomach, which creates fatty acids, which help us to boost iron absorption, which in turn helps to reduce anaemia. Simply drink a glass of water containing a squeeze of lemon juice before each meal.

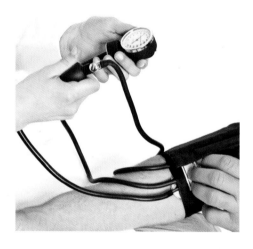

High Blood Pressure

Lemons can be very useful in helping tackle the causes and results of high blood pressure (hypertension). Lemons contain potassium and magnesium and they also promote healthy arteries, whilst their acids discourage insulin resistance.

Just the flavour of a lemon discourages you from adding salt to your food. Salt is often associated with high blood pressure and should be used to a minimum.

Lemon juice also helps release calcium from meat and fish bones, which is valuable in ensuring stable blood-pressure levels.

To be even more scientific, lemon juice operates rather like an ace inhibitor. This simply means it helps decrease the production of a hormone called angiotensin, which has been shown to raise blood pressure by constricting blood vessels.

For generations Russians have used lemons to control blood pressure, and tests in Japan have shown that the consumption of lemon juice has been linked with a reduction in the number of patients with high blood pressure.

High Cholesterol

There are many reasons why you might have high cholesterol, such as insufficient sunlight or exercise or a poor diet. The liver creates most of the body's cholesterol and the lemon can have an impact on how this occurs.

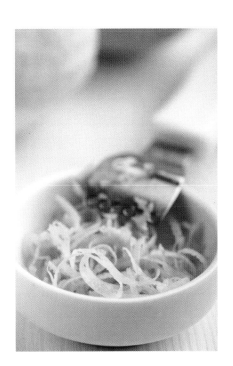

The pectin in a lemon helps to reduce the absorption of cholesterol from food. In the gut pectin also helps inhibit cholesterol absorption. This, together with its Vitamin C, means that the lemon can deliver a double blow against cholesterol.

A lemon is often described as being an alkaline-forming food and research has shown that it does help dissolve and eliminate cholesterol. If you were to eat four apples every day then in terms of cholesterol lowering they would perform the same as a strong statin drug, which is designed to reduce cholesterol. Well, step aside apples, because lemons have more pectin in them, so they are even more effective!

Immune System Strengthening

The Vitamin C in a lemon is great for improving your overall immunity. Pectin fibre in the lemons stimulates the production of antibodies and white blood cells. They also help create a protein, which deals with inflammation. So making sure that lemons are in your daily diet can certainly help your overall immunity to fight off coughs, colds, infections or viruses.

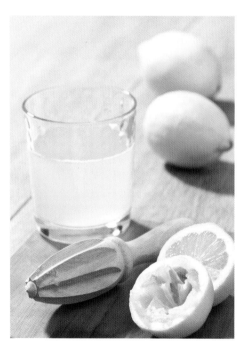

Anti-Inflammatory

The lemon can work as a wonderful anti-inflammatory. Squeeze half a fresh lemon into a glass and add 1 tsp of agave (a natural sweetener from Mexico or South Africa). Alternatively, add 10 drops of stevia, another sweetener and part of the sunflower family. Add a tiny amount of turmeric to taste and top up the glass with spring water. Drink this anti-inflammatory internal cleanser every two hours and drink plenty of water in between each dose.

Arthritis

As lemons are anti-inflammatory, the antioxidant properties of a lemon's peel and juice can help with most types of arthritis. Grate the peel of a lemon and rub this over the aching joint. Make sure that you do not apply the pith. Wrap the joint after applying the lemon peel with a bandage and leave it for at least two hours.

Alternatively, squeeze half a lemon into a small amount of almond oil and massage the painful joint.

It is also possible to relieve painful joints by drinking the juice of a whole lemon in a glass of warm water each day.

Gout

Drinking the juice of a lemon in some warm water can help gout sufferers. Gout is caused by uric acid in the blood and tissue. This acid crystallizes in the joints, causing intense pain. The juice of a lemon can encourage the body to create calcium carbonate, which neutralizes uric acid.

Joint and Nerve Pain

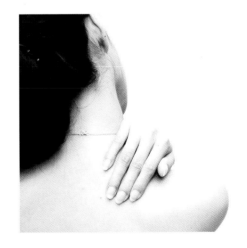

Lemon juice has anti-inflammatory and cooling properties, so it is ideal for applying directly to troublesome joints and painful limbs, including areas that might be suffering from neuralgia. The simple solution is to warm the juice of a lemon and apply it directly to the affected area. Repeat the treatment each hour for at least half a day.

As an alternative you could try putting three drops of lemon oil into a little almond oil and using this as a massage oil for the affected area.

Neuralgia

Neuralgia can be very painful and once again the anti-inflammatory properties of the lemon can come to the rescue. Ideally you should use warm lemon juice, so pop a lemon into the microwave for 30 seconds, cut it in half and squeeze out the juice. This heating process will also encourage more juice to be released from the lemon. Rub the lemon juice onto the area affected by the neuralgia and repeat this as often as you need to reduce the pain.

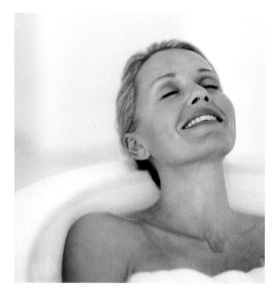

Anxiety and Stress

If you are suffering from anxiety, the simplest and most irritating thing that people can tell you to do is to relax. But it is good advice, and lemons can help.

Bizarrely, the solution is to pour a cup of tea into a hot bath. The bath needs to be as hot as you can bear, but before clambering in, you need to put two lemon tea bags into a bowl. Half fill the bowl with hot water, add a dash of milk and then squeeze in the juice from a whole lemon. Pour this mixture into your bath and gently relax for at least 30 minutes.

Stress, which is often the cause of anxiety, can also be tackled by either improving your consumption of Vitamin C, or by using lemon oil to alleviate the symptoms. To increase your Vitamin C intake squeeze the juice of a lemon into a glass, top up with water and drink first thing daily. Alternatively, have a paper tissue handy and soak up a couple of drops of lemon oil. Inhale whenever you feel stress overtaking you.

Depression

Inhaling the vapour from lemon oil is believed by some psychologists to help ease depression. Simply put a few drops of lemon oil into a diffuser. Alternatively, if you do not have lemon oil readily available, put a few drops of lemon juice onto a paper tissue and inhale it from time to time.

Fainting and Fatigue

A lemon's acidity and fibre should slow down the absorption of sugar from the gut. This in turn helps prevent high blood sugar and then low blood sugar, which is often the cause of fainting.

Adding lemon juice and zest to your daily diet can help eliminate dizzy spells. Many people who use up their blood sugar quickly often feel faint after eating, so acidic foods help to promote the digestion of the food's proteins.

For fatigue, the fibre in a lemon helps to slow down sugar absorption. Lemons are packed with vitamins, and they contain some Vitamin B, which is good at alleviating fatigue. If you tend to get really tired make sure you are including some lemon juice and zest in your daily diet, too.

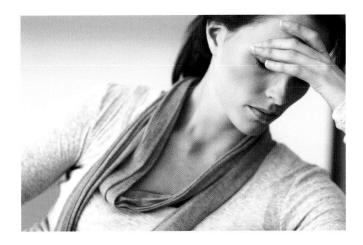

Insomnia

Relaxation and calming the brain are the keys to having a restful night's sleep. The simple solution is to drink lemon tea as your last beverage of the night.

Alternatively you can inhale the vapour from lemon oil, which is believed to have sedative properties. You can always drop some lemon oil into the bath before bedtime.

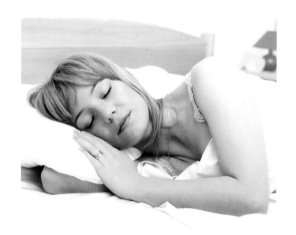

A slightly more complex way of dealing with insomnia is to mix a few drops of lemon oil, ylang ylang oil and vetivert oil together. The ylang ylang is believed to be an anti-depressant and the vetivert a comforting sedative. Massage your stomach with this oil mix before getting into bed. Some people also swear by putting a few drops of lemon oil onto their pillow.

You could also try mixing 2 tsp of lemon juice with 2 tbsp of honey and combining this in a cup of warm milk. Warming the milk activates the natural tryptophan the liquid contains and this induces sleep. Drink this warm, lemony milk drink about 30 minutes before bedtime.

Vitamin C Deficiency

The most extreme case of Vitamin C deficiency is one that used to afflict mariners in the past – scurvy. This presented itself as thinning hair, dry, flaky skin, fatigue and bleeding gums. The solution was to drink lemon or lime juice every day. Lemon juice is one of the best sources of Vitamin C.

Humans are one of the few animals that are unable to make their own Vitamin C, and the exact amount of Vitamin C that your body needs depends on your age and general health. Vitamin C is vital to help with cardiovascular and joint problems and cataracts, which are associated with Vitamin C deficiency. Vitamin C acts as an antioxidant and prevents oxygen-based damage to cells. Many of our cells are dependent on Vitamin C for protection. A deficiency will show itself if you become susceptible to colds and infections, as well as having a generally weak immune system. You may also become susceptible to respiratory infections and lung problems.

Lemon juice also has flavonoids, which are powerful antioxidants that fight the ageing process and help us to fight disease.

Asthma

In addition to your inhaler, there are several ways in which lemon juice can be used to help ease asthma and prevent asthma attacks – the anti-inflammatory antioxidants in the lemon can come to the rescue if you have inflamed or sensitive airways.

Squeeze the juice of half a lemon and drink this with a little water two or three times a day. This will help prevent asthma attacks as it reduces the inflammation of the airway.

If you are suffering from an asthma attack, squeeze a little lemon juice into a glass of water and sip it over the course of the next 30 minutes. Wait for another 30 minutes and repeat.

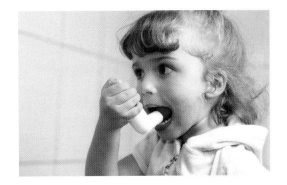

Some asthma sufferers swear by pure lemon juice. They take half a spoonful before each meal and another before they go to bed.

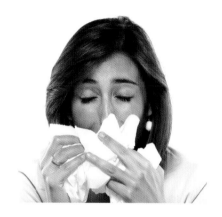

Another option is to prepare a strong lemon solution. Squeeze the juice of a whole lemon into a cup and add boiling water and some honey to taste. Sip the drink whilst you inhale the steam.

Hay Fever

Lemons have anti-inflammatory and antihistamine properties, which can both help to discourage hay fever or allergic reactions. If you have hay fever you could try squeezing the juice of half a lemon into a glass of water. You should drink three of these lemony drinks during the course of the day. If the hay fever or allergy has given you a sore throat then gargle the mixture, but this time use warm water.

Bronchitis

Lemon juice is packed with Vitamin C and citric acid, so it is ideal for helping to deal with chest complaints such as bronchitis. When you have bronchitis it is best to drink plenty of fluids, as this helps get rid of the mucous. Lemon juice, particularly if taken with a little warm water, will also soothe an irritating cough.

To also aid your breathing, squeeze the juice of a lemon into a bowl of steaming hot water. Cover your head with a towel and breathe in the steam. For extra relief add a few drops of eucalyptus, peppermint or rosemary oil, as these will also help to clear your airways and soothe the irritation.

Coughs

The oil in lemons can help expel mucous, so to soothe a cough you could make your own home-made lemonade (*see* page 144) and drink it daily.

Alternatively, slice half a lemon and use a pestle and mortar to break up 2 tbsp of linseeds. Put these into 600 ml/1 pint/2½ cups of water and simmer in a pan for 20 minutes. Strain and add honey to sweeten the mixture.

Another option is to boil up a bowl of water and add two drops each of lemon oil, eucalyptus oil and tea-tree oil. Put a towel over your head and inhale.

A further home-made cough remedy is to heat 4 tbsp of lemon juice, 180 ml/6 fl oz/scant ¾ cup of honey and 6 tbsp of olive oil. Stir the mixture whilst heating. Allow it to cool and then take 1 tsp of the mixture every two or three hours for the next 48 hours.

Sore Throat

Gargling is the solution for a sore throat. You will need to squeeze the juice of one lemon into a small amount of hot water. If you gargle three times a day with this mixture the soreness will subside as the lemon juice gets to work on the damaged areas of your throat and tackles the inflammation.

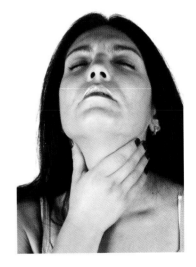

Bad Breath

Lemons can be used as a mouthwash, as the juice is a great antiseptic. Squeeze the juice of a lemon into a glass and gargle with it. If you are feeling brave you can swallow the juice, or alternatively spit out and rinse the mouth. The citric acid kills off the bacteria in your mouth and alters the pH level of the body.

CAUTION: Do not gargle with lemon juice in your mouth for too long as it can affect the enamel on the teeth.

Hangovers

Hangovers can give you a headache, they can make you feel dehydrated and sometimes nauseous. For the headache you can rub a slice of lemon on your temple and forehead, or squeeze half a lemon into a cup of strong, black coffee. Alternatively, squeeze the juice of half a lemon onto a tissue and inhale.

For the hangover, and to give you a perk up, cut a lemon into quarter wedges and then sprinkle each quarter with salt. Brace yourself as you then eat the pulp, but not the pith or rind. This is guaranteed to wake you up!

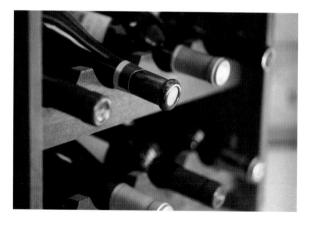

Some people believe that prevention is far better than a cure. So if you have had a heavy night then squeeze the juice of a lemon into a glass of water and drink it before you go to bed. The Vitamin C in the lemon will help break down the alcohol in the liver. The lemon juice will also help with rehydration and your Vitamin C levels will be higher when you wake up in the morning.

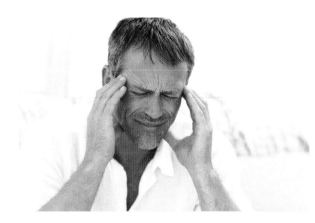

Headaches

We've already seen that a headache brought on by a hangover can easily be dealt with using lemons (*see* page 120). Whether you prefer tea or coffee first thing in the morning, if you have a regular headache just squeeze the juice of a lemon into your first cup.

An alternative for curing a headache with lemons is to sponge your head with the juice of half a lemon in a cup of water. It is also believed that inhaling the vapour from lemon juice can get rid of a headache.

Mouth Ulcers

This is going to sting! But there is no way of avoiding it if you want to get rid of that painful mouth ulcer.

Squeeze the juice of a lemon into a glass of water and gargle with it. The lemon juice will kill off bacteria and disinfect the ulcer. If you are feeling particularly brave there are two more treatments that will guarantee to make you wince.

The first is simple enough. Squeeze out some lemon juice, dip a cotton bud into the juice, brace yourself and apply directly to the ulcer. A slightly milder version uses essential oils. Three drops of tea-tree oil, two of myrrh oil and three of lemon oil are required, with a little almond oil. Apply either with a cotton bud or your clean finger, directly onto the ulcer, at two hourly intervals. This will numb, disinfect and kill bacteria all in one go.

Digestion Aid

Poor digestion can lead to constipation. Lemon juice in hot water, with a little honey added, can be taken each morning to aid the digestive system. Lemons have potassium, minerals and Vitamin C and other natural ingredients, all of which help cleanse the body.

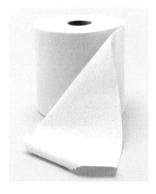

Constipation and Diarrhoea

To help ease constipation, as soon as you get up in the morning, boil the kettle and squeeze the juice of a whole lemon into a mug. Top this juice up with hot water. Make sure you drink it whilst it is still warm, at least 30 minutes before you eat breakfast. Repeat this at night before going to bed.

Lemons can also help in exactly the opposite way, as they are useful in helping to deal with diarrhoea. The pectin in lemons helps to bind the bowel contents and also forms a coating, which soothes irritation. The cellulose in lemons attracts water, which makes the contents of the bowel bulkier.

Lemons are used in West Africa to help protect against cholera, due to the citric acid they contain. The acidity of lemons is very similar to that of stomach acid, so this makes lemons very useful if you do not produce much stomach acid naturally. To help your bowel, make sure you include lemon juice and the zest as part of your daily diet.

Haemorrhoids

Haemorrhoids can be extremely painful and debilitating. The spongy pads can become inflamed, itch and bleed. They can be caused by fragile veins or constipation. The fibre in a lemon helps to prevent constipation and the Vitamin C strengthens the veins. Lemons are also known for their anti-inflammatory antioxidants, which are good for reducing inflammation.

There are two ways of tackling piles with lemon juice. Squeeze the juice of half a lemon into a glass of water and drink it first thing in the morning, before your bathroom visit. At bedtime try mixing ½ tbsp of lemon juice with a similar amount of glycerine, then dab the mixture onto the haemorrhoids each night to help soothe.

Urine Infection

Urinary infections, or cystitis, are painful and can make you feel really miserable. To get rid of it you need to reduce acidifying foods and increase alkalizing foods. Lemons can help with this process. Squeeze the juice of a lemon into a glass of warm water and drink this first thing in the morning. It will change the pH of the urinary tract and discourage the proliferation of bad bacteria, which cause the inflammation of the mucous membranes and walls of the urinary tract.

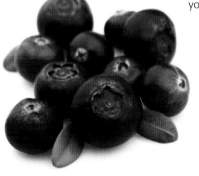

You should make sure that you also drink a lot of filtered water each day. Add cranberries and blueberries to your diet and certainly avoid alcohol, fizzy soft drinks, tomatoes, yeast, sugar and artificial sweeteners. With the exception of the lemon juice you should also avoid other citrus fruits while the infection remains. Believe it or not, the citric acid in the lemon juice will have an alkalizing effect on the urinary tract. It will also reduce inflammation whilst cleansing and cooling, as well as operating as an astringent and antiseptic.

CAUTION: Do not use other citrus fruits, such as oranges or grapefruits, for this treatment, as they do not have the same therapeutic qualities as a lemon.

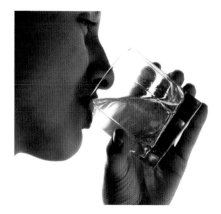

Urine Retention

Squeezing half a lemon into a glass of water is a simple remedy for eliminating fluid retention. Strange though it may seem, in order to prevent water retention you need to drink more water. It is usually the case that the body retains water when we are dehydrated. By drinking up to 10 glasses of water a day most cases of water retention will be eliminated. You should avoid food that has additional sodium, such as salt.

CAUTION: You should not eliminate all sodium from your diet. Switch to fresher food, particularly vegetables, rather than adding salt to the diet.

Cramps

Lemon tea is often taken as a cure for stomach cramps. Some recommend squeezing the juice of a lemon and then infusing a curry leaf, with a pinch of sugar. This can be consumed as an instant relief for stomach pains of all kinds.

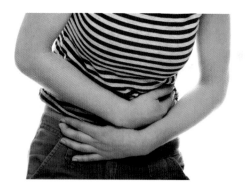

Fibroids

Women with an imbalance of oestrogen and progesterone may often be prone to the growth of womb muscle fibres, known as fibroids. This is also true if an individual is overweight, because fat cells also produce oestrogen.

The fibre in a lemon helps to encourage the re-absorption of oestrogen from the bowel and into the blood and the B vitamins present help the liver to break down the oestrogen. So including the juice and zest of a lemon in a daily diet can have an impact on fibroids.

Stimulating or Suppressing Appetite

Surprisingly, a lemon can help to both stimulate and suppress appetite. Lemon juice and water taken first thing in the morning will reduce and suppress your appetite initially because it fills up the stomach – it also picks you up and makes you feel more alert – but it can also stimulate the appetite, as it stimulates digestion and liver function, as well as detoxifying and cleansing the bowel.

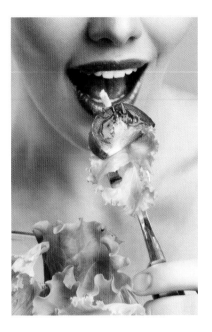

Detox Diets

There are various recipes for a lemon juice detox. Keep any of the following mixtures stored in the refrigerator.

The most well-known recipe is to prepare a cup of hot water and squeeze in the juice of a whole lemon. Add sugar or honey to taste. The lemon juice needs to be taken first thing in the morning and throughout the day you should be sure to consume plenty of water. It is thought that the lemon juice flushes out toxins, particularly from the liver.

In a recipe from the United States cold, filtered water is used, along with 2 tbsp of fresh lemon juice, 2 tbsp of organic maple syrup and a pinch or two of cayenne pepper. This

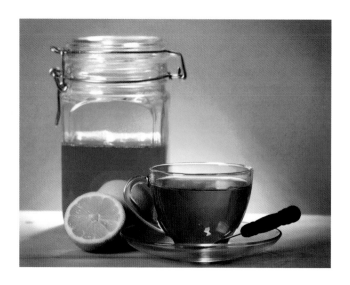

lemon detox diet recommends that 6 to 12 of these servings are consumed every day.

A slightly less extreme version is designed to last for just two days. Mix together 500 ml/18 fl oz/2 cups of lemon juice, 1 litre/1¾ pints/4 cups of orange juice and 1.5 litres/2½ pints/6⅓ cups of grapefruit juice. Water down the mixture to the strength you prefer. Drink one cup every hour until the whole of your two-day mixture has been consumed.

The downside of these detox diets is that you cannot have anything to eat during their duration. It is not recommended that you continue any of these diets for more than seven days.

CAUTION: A lemon detox diet is quite extreme and if taken alone will lead to weight loss.

Metabolic Rate Increase

The lemon detox diet is specifically designed to encourage an increase in the metabolic rate (which measures how quickly your body converts food into energy), to burn up body fat, whilst cleansing, detoxifying and rejuvenating the body.

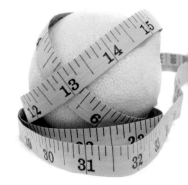

During a lemon detox diet the natural process of ridding the body of toxins continues, but you are not taking any more toxins into your body. At the same time, any energy that you would normally use to digest your food is re-routed to promote cell growth and improve your immune system. As a result the immune system does not need to work as hard as usual and your digestive system is not susceptible to inflammation due to allergic reactions to food. At the same time any chemicals in your system, such as pesticides or drugs, are flushed out.

Gall Stones

Gall stones are formed in the gall bladder by stagnant bile, or calcium salts. They are often associated with diabetes, constipation and obesity and are much more common if you have an unhealthy diet.

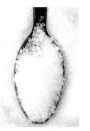

The pectin in a lemon should stop bile acids from the gut being re-absorbed, which helps to prevent gall stones from forming. The lemon juice alone should also encourage the gall bladder to contract and flush out bile and small gall stones.

You can give your gall bladder a thorough flushing by following a fairly extreme, but effective, regime. For six days drink 1 litre/1¾ pints/4 cups of apple juice and on the seventh day take 2 tbsp of Epsom salts in water. Wait one hour and then take 120 ml/4 fl oz/½ cup of olive oil with 4 tbsp of lemon juice. You should then lie on the left side of your body for 30 minutes before going to bed for the night. The theory is that the flush will not only encourage the gall bladder to contract, but it will also soften any gall stones that may be present.

As a less extreme treatment, take 1 tbsp of lemon juice mixed with an equal amount of olive oil an hour before eating each morning. This is thought to help the body break down gall stones, as well as encouraging

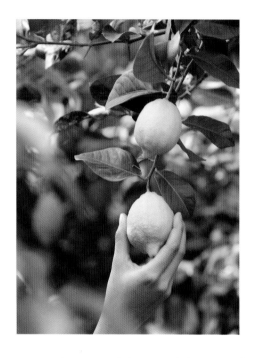

the contraction of the gall bladder. A contracted gall bladder helps expel any gall stones that are present.

If you are prone to gall stones you should certainly consider incorporating at least two lemons in your daily diet.

CAUTION: Always consult your doctor if any painful symptoms persist.

Kidney Stones

Lemon juice is a diuretic, which encourages the production of urine. Lemons also have citric acid, which encourages the liver to create enzymes.

Lemons can help prevent kidney stones from forming, as they provide Vitamin B, fibre, magnesium, calcium and selenium. Lemon juice can also help dissolve existing stones. Some stones are made up of calcium and they are formed because the body fluids are too acidic. The lemon juice has an alkaline effect on the body.

People with raised blood-sugar levels produce additional insulin, particularly after they eat carbohydrates. This makes the kidneys flush out calcium into the urine. The acidity in a lemon helps to prevent this, so as a preventative measure, incorporate lemons into your daily diet.

To help reduce the excruciating pain that can result from the presence of a kidney stone, squeeze the juice of half a lemon into a glass of water. Drink this mixture and repeat every 30 minutes until the pain is reduced.

Heart Palpitations

Heart palpitations are common and often caused by a poor diet, or stress. Physical activity, smoking and anxiety can also be key triggers for heart palpitations, which can give you an increased pulse rate and a thumping feeling in the chest.

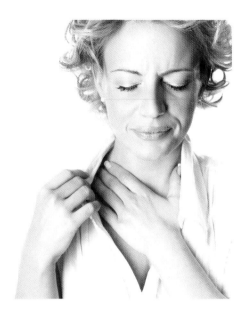

Lemons can again come to the rescue. There are two similar treatments you could try. Squeeze out half a cup of lemon juice and add 1 tbsp of honey. Dilute this mixture with water. Ideally take this mixture before going to bed, but it is also a good general remedy to help you get a feeling of calm.

An alternative is to take the juice of half a lemon and half a lime, along with the honey. Then add 250 ml/8 fl oz/1 cup of water. Take this mixture on a daily basis in order to reduce the likelihood of feeling stressed.

CAUTION: Do not ignore heart palpitations. If they persist contact your doctor.

Heartburn

Citrus fruit juice is not usually recommended as a treatment for heartburn, but diluted lemon juice can help to relieve the burning feeling that some foods can give you. Squeeze the juice of a quarter of a lemon into half a glass of water. Drinking this should alleviate the burning sensation. The lemon juice helps to neutralize gastric acid.

Indigestion

The acids in lemon juice help emulsify fats, particularly those in fried food. This can certainly help prevent indigestion, for people who are prone to it or those that have insufficient stomach acid. This is particularly the case for people over the age of 60 years. By ensuring you include lemons in your daily diet, indigestion can certainly be a thing of the past.

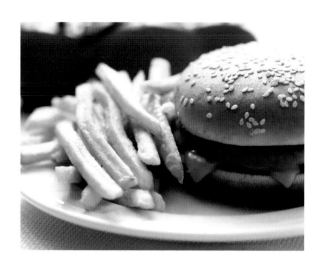

Nausea

Just smelling a lemon can often help reduce that feeling of nausea. Whether it is because of something you have eaten, too much alcohol, or even car sickness, make sure you cut open a lemon and take a deep breath. It should soothe your stomach and get rid of that churning feeling.

Stomach, Liver and Intestines

These are all linked to your metabolic rate (which measures how quickly your body converts food into energy). The thyroid gland determines your metabolic rate. The lemon juice and water mix taken first thing in the morning will certainly get the digestive system working, as well as encouraging liver function. Bitter foods in any case stimulate liver and gall-bladder function. The lemon will also help give your intestines a super clean. Again this is a variation on the lemon detox diet, which incorporates lemon juice, organic maple syrup, a pinch of cayenne pepper and filtered water (*see* page 125). This will help flush through your intestines whilst providing you with a range of vitamins and minerals. You could do the lemon detox diet drink on a daily basis to cleanse the colon.

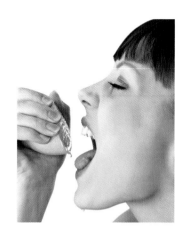

Upset Stomach

Upset stomachs are often associated with an imbalance of the acids contained in the stomach. This can be brought on by an unhealthy diet, where the food that has been consumed encourages the production of acid. In extreme cases poorly digested proteins can be absorbed into the bloodstream, which in turn can cause allergies.

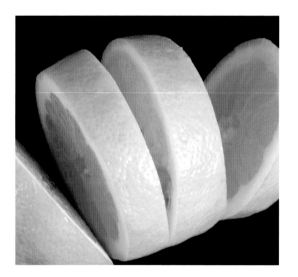

For relief from an upset stomach, try using a lemon. The lemon can help soothe any intestinal pain, relieve constipation and reduce flatulence. Simply squeeze half a lemon into a glass of water and drink this mixture once in the morning and once at night. This will soothe and help the stomach acid return to its normal balance.

Cooking & Recipes

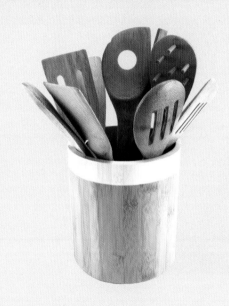

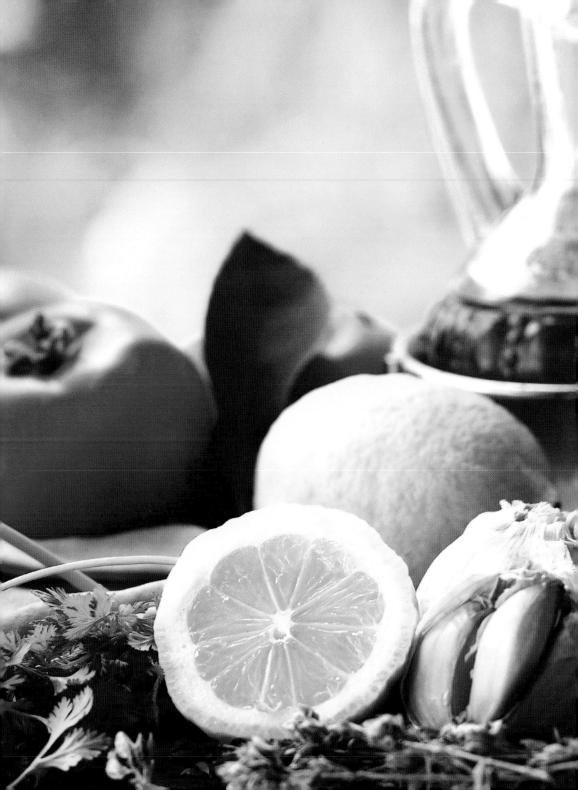

The Basics

The lemon probably ranks third after salt and pepper as the most common and useful culinary ingredient. You can use lemon to bring out the taste of meat and vegetables, to brighten up a dish, to unleash flavours and to make sauces, seasonings and attractive accompaniments. Lemons can be squeezed, peeled, zested or dried. They can even be cooked. The lemon will react with different foods in a host of different ways. They are great for marinades, and for preventing vegetables from losing colour.

Lemon Seasonings

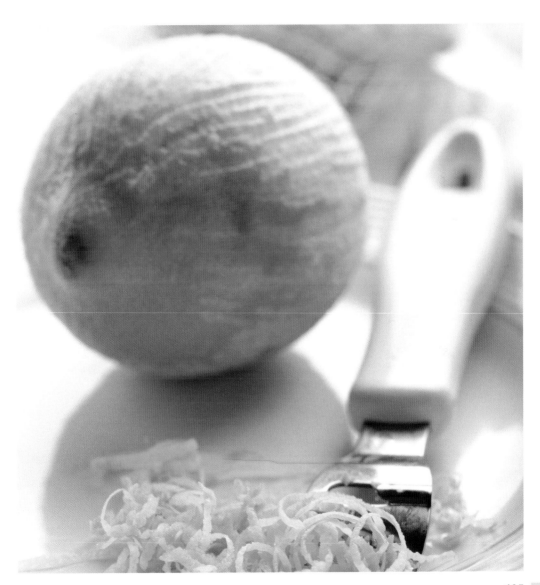

Lemon Zest and Lemon Pepper

You can easily make your own lemon zest, or even pep it up by making a lemon and pepper mix, which is brilliant for seasoning chicken and a host of other foods, as well as being perfect for the barbecue.

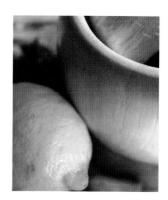

1   Using a zester or a vegetable peeler, remove the yellow zest, taking care not to remove any of the white pith, which can taste sour.

2   When you have removed the zest mince it up and put it into a small bowl.

3   Optionally you can then add two teaspoons of peppercorns. You will need to crack them first with a pestle and mortar, or by putting them onto a cutting board and bashing them with a heavy-based pot or a rolling pin.

4   Mix the zest and cracked pepper together and this will encourage the lemon oils to combine with the pepper.

5   Now spread the zest and pepper onto a baking sheet and leave it in a very low-heat oven overnight to dry out. Or dry it by spreading it on a towel and leaving it until dried.

6   Put the dry mix into a pestle and mortar and pulverize it. Now it is ready to be sprinkled onto your dish, perhaps fish or chicken. To boost the flavour you can squeeze fresh lemon juice over the dish just before cooking. The zest will store well in an airtight jar ' and you can also freeze it.

CAUTION: Unless you are absolutely certain about the source of your lemons, scrub the fruit with a sponge and warm, soapy water before you zest it. This will release any wax or dirt. Rinse well and dry with a paper towel.

Lemon Extract

If you have plenty of time on your hands you can make your own lemon extract. Put the peel of three or four lemons into about 120 ml/4 fl oz/¹⁄₂ cup of water. Place it in a pan and allow it to simmer for a while. Strain the peel, but continue to reduce the liquid to concentrate the flavour. You should get around 2 tbsp of lemony liquid.

Lemon Extract Powder

You can also make lemon extract powder by removing the peel from lemons, making sure that you do not cut off any of the pith. Dry the strips skin-side down on a plate until they are thoroughly dry. This should take about three or four days. Once dry you can pulverize them in a blender, or use a pestle and mortar. Use the powdered peel in a host of different recipes.

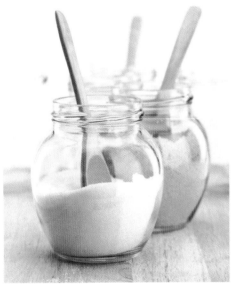

Lemon Sugar

There are two simple ways of making your own lemon sugar. You can use lemon extract powder (see above) and simply add it to the sugar, or you can use lemon twists. Lemon twists are like zested lemon peel, except you use a vegetable peeler to make long strips. Pop some of these twists into a jar with your sugar, and the lemon oil from the peel will infuse into the sugar. Replace the twists when you refill your sugar canister.

Candied Lemon Peel

The tangy flavour of candied lemon peel is so straightforward to make and is a wonderful alternative to confectionery. It is also a brilliant home-made gift, as well as having the added bonus of being fat-free!

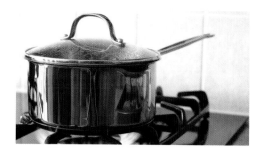

1   Use a knife or citrus peeler to produce long strips of lemon peel. You will probably need to use at least six lemons. Make sure that you try to avoid any of the bitter, white pith.

2   Combine 900 ml/1½ pints/scant 4 cups of water with 2½ cups of sugar. Cook on a medium heat on top of the stove, stirring until the sugar is dissolved. Then allow the mixture to boil for five minutes.

3   Drop in the strips of peel and reduce the heat to a simmer. Continue to cook, but do not stir, until the syrup is reduced to around a quarter. This could take up to two hours.

4   Remove your pan from the heat and allow the liquid to cool before draining the lemon peel. Preheat your oven up to 200°C/400°F/Gas Mark 6.

5   Carefully retrieve each of the peels, one by one, and dunk them into a bowl of sugar. You need to ensure that each one is fully coated.

6   Place the peels on a baking sheet lined with baking parchment. Allow the sugar-coated peels to dry out in the hot oven, which will take around an hour. Make sure you check to ensure that they are not burning.

7   When the peels are completely dry you can scrape off any excess sugar. They should now keep for around a week. As a special treat, why not try dipping the candied peel into melted chocolate!

Preserved Lemons

Salting lemons can take away much
of their sourness and you can then
store them in oil.

You will need:
around 15 small lemons (unwaxed)
3 tbsp salt
2 tbsp paprika
4 bay leaves
720 ml/24 fl oz/3 cups hazelnut or walnut oil

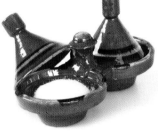
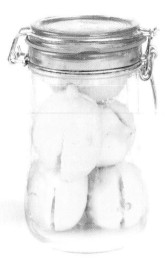

1 Wash and slice the lemons, then
   layer them in a colander and
   sprinkle salt on each layer.
   Leave the lemons for 24 hours and dry them with a paper towel.

2 Prepare a preserving jar by sterilizing it first by putting it in a hot oven for at least
   10 minutes.

3 Begin filling the jar with the slices of lemon. Each layer should have a sprinkle of paprika.
   Every three or four layers add a bay leaf.

4 When you have finished layering the lemons cover with the oil and seal the jar. Store it
   in a cool, dark place.

You can use the lemons immediately, but once the jar is opened it should be stored in a
refrigerator. The lemons should be fine for the next six months.

Alternatively you could store the unopened jar for around two years. These preserved
lemons are wonderful in stews and they make great holiday gifts.

Culinary Tips

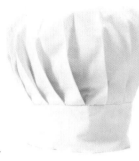

Soften Brown Sugar

Add lemon peel, making sure that you have removed the pith and all of the pulp, to brown sugar. It will keep the sugar moist and easier to use or blend.

Keep Guacamole Green

Have you ever noticed that when you cut or mash an avocado to make guacamole it begins to turn brown very quickly? The same can be said about cut apples, bananas or pears. Sprinkling some fresh lemon juice over the fruit will keep it fresh and green for much longer and the lemon juice will only add to the taste of your guacamole.

Preserve and Marinade Meat

The citric acid in lemon juice can change the pH of meat, which could make it a more hostile environment for bacteria. Applying lemon juice to raw meat could help preserve it.

If you have tough, chewy meat then you can marinade it in lemon juice overnight. The juice will break down muscle tissue, making the meat much more tender. The flavour-enhancing lemon will also add to any meat dish, especially those using chicken or lamb. Try using a marinade of lemon juice, olive oil and oregano next time you barbecue some meat.

Make Sour Milk

To make sour milk or sour cream simply squeeze a little lemon juice into fresh milk or cream.

Whip Cream

You know how sometimes whipping cream just will not whip? Try adding a few drops of lemon juice to solve the problem.

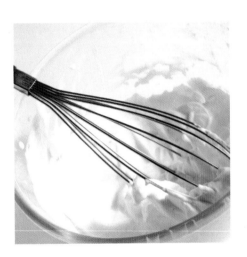

Prevent Sticky Rice

Interestingly, lemon juice, when added to the water when you are cooking rice, makes the rice fluffy and also helps prevent grains from sticking together and clogging.

Prevent Fruit and Vegetables from Turning Brown

As soon as we cut vegetables such as potatoes, sweet potatoes, parsnips, and artichokes, or fruits such as apples, pears and bananas, they start to turn brown. This is because enzymes in their cells are exposed to and react with the oxygen in the air. Simply squeeze a little lemon juice over vegetables or freshly cut fruit while you are preparing them and they will retain their original, vibrant colour.

If you are into making smoothies you may have noticed exactly the same browning problem. It look less appetizing, even though it may still taste delicious. Just add a few drops of lemon juice into the smoothie-maker or electric juicer for all the original colours to be retained.

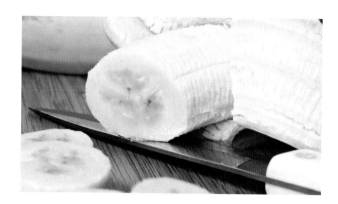

Keep Lettuce Crisp

Lemon juice can be used to stop a lettuce from going limp or from browning after you've cut it. To revive your lettuce drop it into a bowl of cold water that has had the juice of half a lemon added. Pop the bowl into your refrigerator for an hour and the lettuce will recover and be fresh and crispy again.

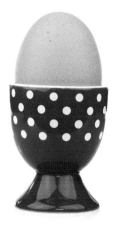

Stop Boiled Eggs from Cracking

If you dab egg shells with lemon juice before you pop them into boiling water then the shells should not crack. To be doubly sure you could also add some more lemon juice to the boiling water. This will also make it easier to peel the eggs.

Crisp the Skin of Poultry Dishes

Whether it be chicken or duck, rub a lemon over the skin before you begin cooking your dish. This will help to ensure that your poultry has delicious, crispy skin.

Make Perfect Poached Eggs

To make sure that your poached eggs are perfect, squeeze a few drops of lemon juice into the boiling water. Swirl the water around and then drop in the eggs.

Enhance the Flavour of Mushrooms

The natural, earthy taste of mushrooms is enhanced by squeezing a little lemon juice over them as they cook. This works regardless of the method of cooking you are using.

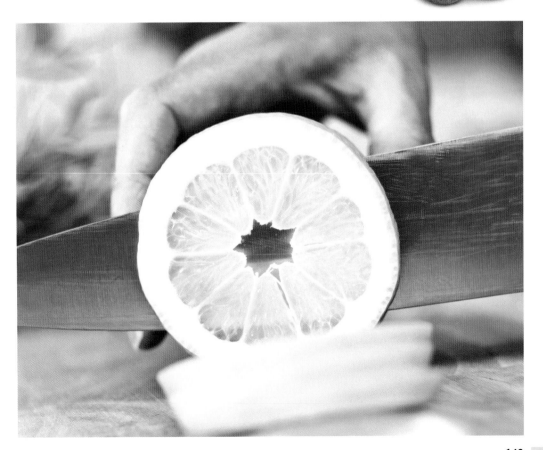

Basic Recipes

Lemonade

There are two ways of making lemonade. One is slightly sweeter than the other.

You will need:

3 lemons, pips removed, sliced
100 g/3^1/$_2$ oz/^{1}/$_2$ cup caster/superfine sugar
2 x 570 ml/20 fl oz/2^1/$_4$ cups boiled water

1   Put the lemon, sugar and the first batch of boiled water into a blender and blitz until smooth.

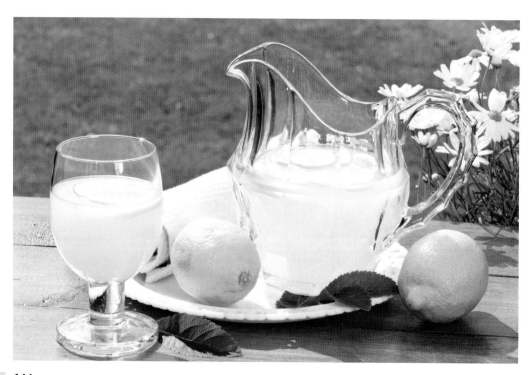

2   Then stir in the second batch of boiled water. Strain into a jug/pitcher. You can drink it warm or pop it in the refrigerator and add ice cubes just before serving.

If you do not have a blender then put the lemon slices and sugar directly into the jug. Add all the boiled water at the same time, which should have just finished boiling. Stir the mixture with a wooden spoon until all the sugar is dissolved, squashing the lemon slices on the side of the jug to make sure you have released all the flavour. Strain the lemonade into a second jug.

If you prefer a less bitter lemon taste, follow the same steps, but this time zest the three lemons and squeeze the juice out of them, rather than slicing them, and discard the pith.

Lemon Barley Water

This is similar to the lemonade recipes above (see page 144).

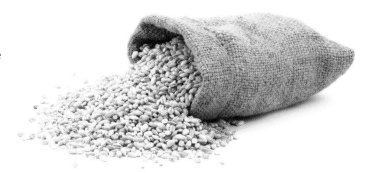

You will need:
1.7 litres/3 pints/7 cups boiled water
75g /3 oz/^{1}/$_3$ cup pearl or wild barley
3 lemons, chopped
50 g/2 oz/^{1}/$_4$ cup sugar

1   Put the water and barley into a pan and bring it to the boil. Cover the pan and allow the mixture to simmer for half an hour.

2   Drop in the lemons and sugar and stir to dissolve the sugar before allowing the whole mixture to cool down.

3   Once it has cooled sufficiently strain it into a jug. Store your lemon barley water in the refrigerator, where it should last for up to five days.

As an alternative, you can use 150 g/5 oz/$^3/_4$ cup of pearl barley, the grated zest and juice of two lemons, 165 g/5$^1/_2$ oz/$^1/_2$ cup of honey and 1.5 litres/2$^1/_2$ pints/6$^1/_3$ cups of water. First rinse the barley in a sieve and then pour the water, lemon zest and barley into a pan. Bring the mixture to a boil and allow it to simmer for 10 minutes before straining it into a bowl. Now add the honey and stir until it is fully dissolved before stirring in the lemon juice. For an additional kick, finely grate a tablespoonful of fresh ginger and add it at the beginning of the process.

Lemon Sorbet

Lemon sorbet is exceptionally good for cleansing the palate. It is also a really easy dessert, as long as you have enough time to wait for it to set in the freezer. You can make your own lemon sorbet, with or without limoncello (an Italian lemon vodka). You can also add your own, special ingredients – even champagne for an extra special occasion!

You will need:
570 ml/20 fl oz/2$^1/_4$ cups water
25 g/80 oz/2 tbsp caster/superfine sugar
5 or 6 lemons (juice only, plus the peel from just 3 of them)
2 tbsp limoncello (optional)
2 egg whites

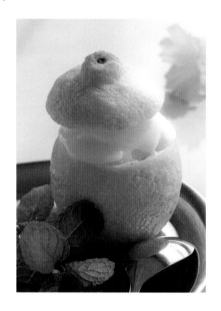

1   Pour the water into a pan and add the sugar. Cook on a medium heat until the sugar is dissolved.

2   Drop in the peel from 3 of your lemons and allow the mixture to simmer for 10 minutes before removing the peel.

3   Pour in the lemon juice and the limoncello, (if using) then pour the whole mixture into a freezable container.

4   Once it is cool, freeze it for 2 hours. The mixture should now be mushy and not frozen solid. Take a fork, stir up the partially frozen mixture.

5   Whisk the egg whites, making sure they form firm peaks.

6   Fold the egg whites into the sorbet thoroughly and put the container back into the freezer for around 4 hours. Take the container out of the freezer for around 30 minutes before serving.

For that added wow factor, why not serve your lemon sorbet in lemons? Just cut off the top third of the lemon, which will become the lid. Hollow out the lemon and the lid and cut a small slice out of the bottom of each lemon so it can stand upright. Put the lemons and the lids in the freezer and after a couple of hours they should harden up. When you are ready to serve the sorbet take them out, fill them with the sorbet, replace the lid and hey presto, no washing-up!

Lemon Curd

Lemon curd is a useful addition to a number of recipes.

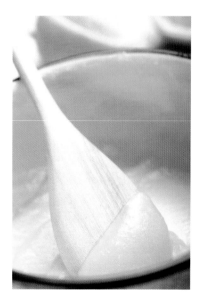

You will need:
125 g/4 oz /¹/₂ cup (1 stick) unsalted butter
juice and zest of 3 lemons
220 g/7 oz/heaping 1 cup of caster/superfine sugar
6 egg yolks

1   Melt the butter in a saucepan and whisk in the lemon juice, zest and sugar.

2   Add the egg yolks and whisk until the mixture is smooth. Continue to heat and stir for up to 15 minutes. You are looking for a consistency that will coat your wooden spoon, but do not allow it to boil.

3   Remove the mixture from the heat and pour into a sterilized preserving jar. Allow the
     mixture to cool in the jar to room temperature and then store it in the refrigerator. You can
     also put the lemon curd into a plastic container and store it in the freezer for two months.

Hot Lemon Punch

This is a great winter warmer that combines red wine, tea, orange, lemon, honey, sugar and spices.

You will need:
1.1 litres/2 pints/4²/₃ cups boiled water
2 tea bags
juice and zest of 1 lemon and 1 orange
1 cinnamon stick
3 cloves
570 ml/20 fl oz/2¹/₄ cups of red wine
1 tbsp sugar (you may wish to add more to taste if you
    have a sweet tooth)
2 tbsp honey

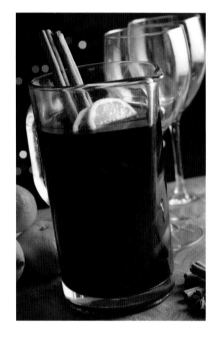

1   Take a large pan and pour in the water and drop in
     the tea bags. Allow the tea bags to infuse for
     around 30 minutes.

2   Take out the tea bags and drop in the lemon and
     orange zest and juice, along with the cloves and
     cinnamon stick. Stir well and allow this to infuse
     for around 30 minutes before adding the wine,
     sugar and honey.

3   Heat the mixture until you get a rolling boil, by which time the honey and sugar
     should have dissolved. Do a test taste and add additional sugar at this stage if you feel
     it is necessary.

Lemon Salad Dressing

One of the simplest salad dressings takes full advantage of the sensation of tangy, fresh lemon.

You will need:
2 tbsp lemon juice
1 tsp mustard powder
a little honey
6 tbsp olive oil
salt and pepper

Combine all of the ingredients in a jar and give it a vigorous shake. You can also add freshly chopped herbs of your choice: basil, parsley, thyme or oregano work perfectly. Your salad dressing is now ready to annoint your salad.

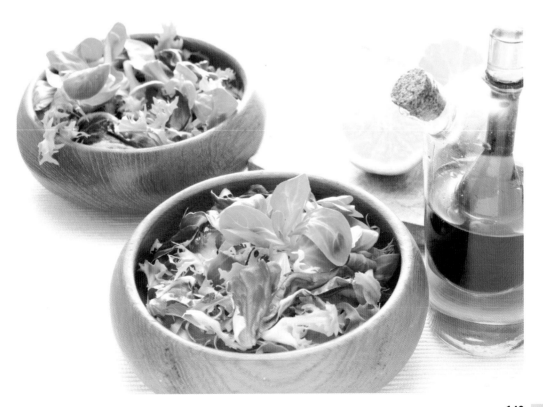

Savoury Dishes

Lemons work brilliantly with a huge range of savoury dishes, from pork to chicken and fish to vegetables. Lemons give a fantastic zing by either using the juice or peel, or both. For generations the lemon has been an important part of many Mediterranean and Middle Eastern dishes. Try out the zingy selection of recipes provided in this section.

Bulgur Wheat Salad with Minty Lemon Dressing

Serves 4

125 g/4½ oz/¾ cup bulgur wheat
125 g/4½ oz/1 cup baby sweetcorn
3 ripe but firm tomatoes
10 cm/4 inch piece cucumber, diced
2 shallots, peeled and finely chopped

For the dressing:

grated rind of 1 lemon
3 tbsp lemon juice
3 tbsp freshly chopped mint
2 tbsp freshly chopped parsley
1–2 tsp clear honey
2 tbsp sunflower oil
salt and freshly ground black pepper

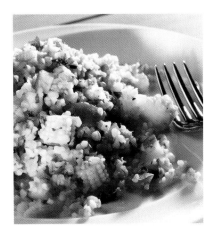

1   Place the bulgur wheat in a saucepan and cover with boiling water. Simmer for about 10 minutes, then drain thoroughly and turn into a serving bowl.

2   Steam the baby sweetcorn over a pan of boiling water for 10 minutes, or until tender. Drain and slice into thick chunks.

3   Cut a cross on the top of each tomato and place in boiling water until their skins start to peel away. Remove the skins and the seeds and cut the tomatoes into small cubes.

4   Make the dressing by briskly whisking all the ingredients in a small bowl until well mixed. When the bulgur wheat has cooled a little, add all the prepared vegetables and stir in the dressing. Season to taste with salt and pepper and serve.

Pasta with Courgettes, Rosemary & Lemon

Serves 4

50 g/2 oz/4/½ cups dried pasta shapes, e.g. rigatoni
1½ tbsp good-quality extra virgin olive oil
2 garlic cloves, peeled and finely chopped
4 medium courgettes/zucchini, thinly sliced
1 tbsp freshly chopped rosemary
1 tbsp freshly chopped parsley
zest and juice of 2 lemons
2 tbsp roughly chopped pitted black/ripe olives
2 tbsp roughly chopped pitted green olives
salt and freshly ground
black pepper

To garnish:

lemon slices
sprigs of fresh rosemary

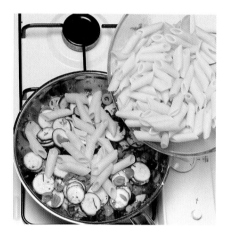

1   Bring a large saucepan of salted water to the boil and add the pasta. Return to the boil and cook until al dente or according to the packet instructions.

2   Meanwhile, when the pasta is almost done, heat the oil in a large frying pan and add the garlic. Cook over a medium heat until the garlic just begins to brown. Be careful not to overcook the garlic at this stage or it will become bitter.

3   Add the courgettes/zucchini, rosemary, parsley and lemon zest and juice. Cook for 3–4 minutes until the courgettes are just tender.

4   Add the olives to the frying pan and stir well. Season to taste with salt and pepper and remove from the heat.

5   Drain the pasta well and add to the frying pan. Stir until thoroughly combined. Garnish with lemon and sprigs of fresh rosemary and serve immediately.

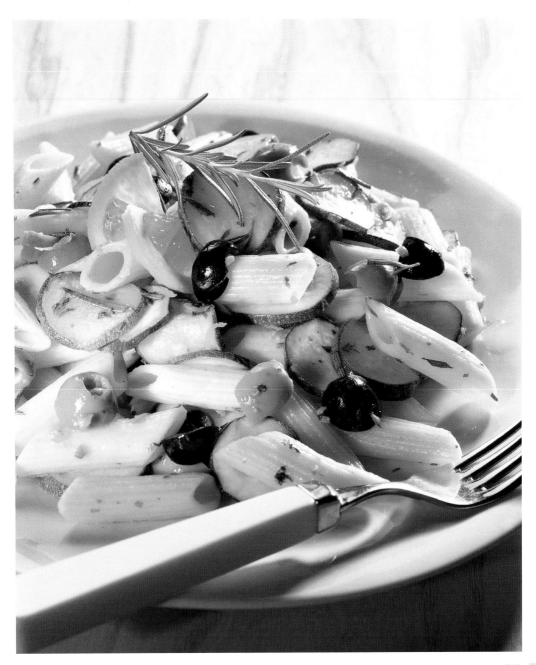

Griddled Garlic & Lemon Squid

Serves 4

25 g/4 oz long-grain rice
300 ml/½ pint/1¼ cups fish stock
225 g/8 oz squid, cleaned
finely grated rind of 1 lemon
1 garlic clove, peeled and crushed
1 shallot, peeled and finely chopped
2 tbsp freshly chopped coriander/cilantro
2 tbsp lemon juice
salt and freshly ground black pepper

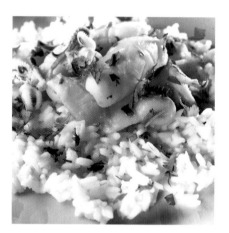

1   Rinse the rice until the water runs clear, then place in a saucepan with the stock. Bring to the boil, then reduce the heat. Cover and simmer gently for 10 minutes. Turn off the heat and leave the pan covered so the rice can steam while you cook the squid.
2   Remove the tentacles from the squid and reserve.
3   Cut the body cavity in half. Using the tip of a small sharp knife, score the inside flesh of the body cavity in a diamond pattern. Do not cut all the way through.
4   Mix the lemon rind, crushed garlic and chopped shallot together.
5   Place the squid in a shallow bowl and sprinkle over the lemon mixture and stir.
6   Heat a griddle pan/ridged grill pan until almost smoking. Cook the squid for 3–4 minutes until cooked through, then slice.
7   Sprinkle with the coriander/cilantro and lemon juice. Season to taste with salt and pepper. Drain the rice and serve immediately with the squid.

Seared Salmon & Lemon Linguine

Serves 4

4 small skinless salmon fillets, each about 75 g/3 oz
2 tsp sunflower oil
½ tsp crushed mixed or black peppercorns
400 g/14 oz linguine
15 g/½ oz/1 tbsp unsalted butter
1 bunch spring onions/scallions, trimmed and shredded
300 ml/½ pint/1¼ cups sour cream
zest of 1 lemon, finely grated
50 g/2 oz/½ cup freshly grated Parmesan cheese
1 tbsp lemon juice
pinch salt

To garnish:

dill sprigs
lemon slices

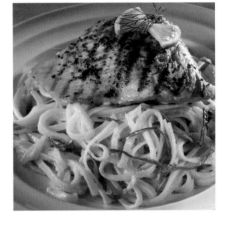

1   Brush the salmon fillets with the sunflower oil, sprinkle with crushed peppercorns and press on firmly and reserve.
2   Bring a large pan of lightly salted water to a rolling boil. Add the linguine and cook according to the packet instructions, or until al dente.
3   Meanwhile, melt the butter in a saucepan and cook the shredded spring onions/scallions gently for 2–3 minutes, or until soft. Stir in the sour cream and the lemon zest and remove from the heat.
4   Preheat a griddle pan/ridged grill pan or heavy-based frying pan until very hot. Add the salmon and sear for 1½–2 minutes on each side. Remove from the pan and allow to cool slightly.
5   Bring the sour cream sauce to the boil and stir in the Parmesan cheese and lemon juice. Drain the pasta thoroughly and return to the pan. Pour over the sauce and toss gently to coat. Spoon the pasta on to warmed serving plates and top with the salmon fillets. Serve immediately with dill sprigs and lemon slices.

Lemon Chicken Rice

Serves 4

2 tbsp sunflower oil
4 chicken leg portions
1 medium onion, peeled and chopped
1–2 garlic cloves, peeled and crushed
1 tbsp curry powder
25 g/1 oz/2 tbsp butter
225 g/8 oz/1⅓ cups long-grain white rice
1 lemon, preferably unwaxed, sliced
600 ml/1 pint/2½ cups chicken stock
salt and freshly ground black pepper
2 tbsp flaked, toasted almonds
sprigs of fresh coriander/cilantro, to garnish

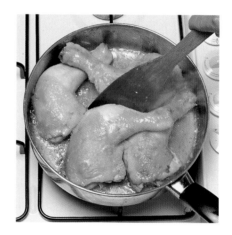

1   Preheat the oven to 180°C/ 350°F/Gas Mark 4, about 10 minutes before required. Heat the oil in a large frying pan, add the chicken legs and cook, turning, until sealed and golden all over. Using a slotted spoon, remove from the pan and reserve.

2   Add the onion and garlic to the oil remaining in the frying pan and cook for 5–7 minutes, or until just beginning to brown. Sprinkle in the curry powder and cook, stirring, for a further 1 minute. Return the chicken to the pan and stir well, then remove from the heat.

3   Melt the butter in a large heavy-based saucepan. Add the rice and cook, stirring, to ensure that all the grains are coated in the melted butter, then remove from the heat.

4   Stir the lemon slices into the chicken mixture, then spoon the mixture onto the rice and pour over the stock. Season to taste with salt and pepper. Cover with an airtight lid and cook in the preheated oven for 45 minutes or until the rice is tender and the chicken is cooked thoroughly. Serve sprinkled with the toasted flaked almonds, and sprigs of coriander/cilantro.

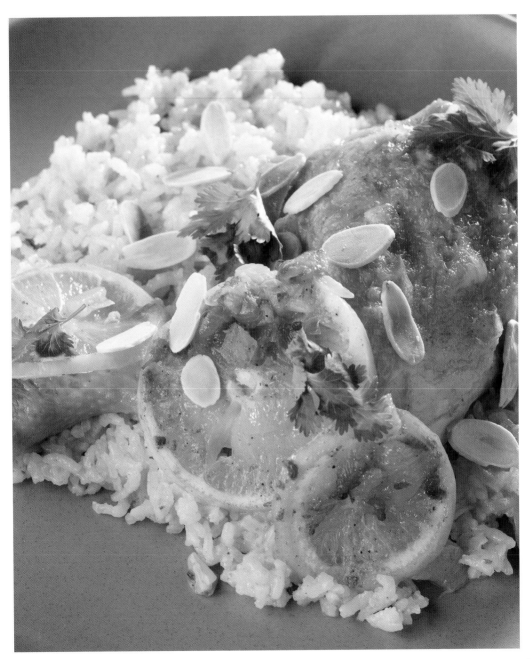

Lemon Chicken with Potatoes, Rosemary & Olives

Serves 6

12 skinless, boneless chicken thighs
1 large lemon
125 ml/4 fl oz/$\frac{1}{2}$ cup extra virgin olive oil
6 garlic cloves, peeled and sliced
2 onions, peeled and thinly sliced
bunch fresh rosemary
1.1 kg/2$\frac{1}{2}$ lb (about 5 medium) potatoes,
    peeled and cut into 4 cm/1$\frac{1}{2}$ inch pieces
salt and freshly ground black pepper
18–24 black olives, pitted

To serve:

steamed carrots
steamed courgettes/zucchini

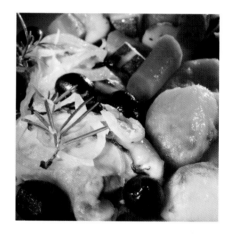

1   Preheat oven to 200°C/400°F/Gas Mark 6, 15 minutes before baking. Trim the chicken thighs and place in a shallow baking dish large enough to hold them in a single layer.

2   Remove the zest from the lemon with a zester or, if using a peeler, cut into thin julienne strips. Reserve half and add the remainder to the chicken. Squeeze the lemon juice over the chicken, toss to coat well and leave to stand for 10 minutes. Add the remaining lemon zest or julienne strips, olive oil, garlic, onions and half of the rosemary sprigs. Toss gently and leave for about 20 minutes.

3   Cover the potatoes with lightly salted water and bring to the boil. Cook for 2 minutes, then drain well and add to the chicken. Season to taste with salt and pepper. Roast the chicken in the preheated oven for 50 minutes, turning frequently and basting, or until the chicken is cooked.

4   Just before the end of cooking time, discard the rosemary and add fresh rosemary sprigs. Add the olives and stir. Serve immediately with steamed carrots and courgettes/zucchini.

Lemon Chicken with Basil & Linguine

Serves 4

grated zest and juice of 1 large lemon
2 garlic cloves, peeled and crushed
2 tbsp basil-flavoured extra virgin olive oil
4 tbsp freshly chopped basil
salt and freshly ground black pepper
450 g/1 lb skinless, boneless chicken breast,
   cut into bite-size pieces
1 onion, peeled and finely chopped
3 celery stalks, trimmed and thinly sliced
175 g/6 oz/1¹⁄₂ cups wiped and halved mushrooms
2 tbsp plain/all-purpose flour
150 ml/¹⁄₄ pint/²⁄₃ cup white wine
150 ml/¹⁄₄ pint/²⁄₃ cup chicken stock
350–450 g/12 oz–1 lb/4–6 cups linguine

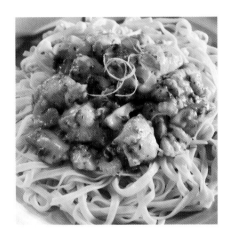

To garnish:

lemon zest and fresh basil leaves

1   Blend the lemon zest and juice, garlic, half the oil, half the basil and salt and pepper in a large bowl. Add the chicken and toss well. Allow to stand for about 1 hour, stirring occasionally.

2   Heat the remaining oil in a large nonstick frying pan, then add the onion and cook for 3–4 minutes until slightly softened. Using a slotted spoon, drain the chicken pieces and add to the frying pan, reserving the marinade. Cook the chicken for 2–3 minutes until golden brown, then add the celery and mushrooms and cook for a further 2–3 minutes.

3   Sprinkle in the flour and stir until the chicken and vegetables are coated. Gradually stir in the wine until a thick sauce forms, then stir in the stock and reserved marinade. Bring to the boil, stirring constantly. Cover and simmer for about 10 minutes, then stir in the remaining basil.

4   Meanwhile, bring a large saucepan of lightly salted water to the boil, add the linguine and simmer for 7–10 minutes until *al dente*. Drain well and turn into a large serving bowl, pour over the sauce and garnish with the lemon zest and fresh basil leaves. Serve immediately.

Stir-Fried Lemon Chicken

Serves 4

350 g/12 oz skinless, boneless chicken breast
1 large/extra-large egg white
5 tsp cornflour/cornstarch
3 tbsp vegetable or groundnut/peanut oil
150 ml/$^1/_4$ pint/$^2/_3$ cup chicken stock
2 tbsp fresh lemon juice
2 tbsp light soy sauce
1 tbsp Chinese rice wine or dry sherry
1 tbsp sugar
2 garlic cloves, peeled and finely chopped
$^1/_4$ tsp dried chilli flakes, or to taste

To garnish:

lemon rind strips
red chilli slices

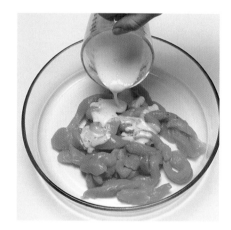

1   Using a sharp knife, trim the chicken, discarding any fat, and cut into thin strips, about 5 cm/2 inches long and 1 cm/$^1/_2$ inch wide. Place in a shallow dish. Lightly whisk the egg white and 1 tablespoon of the cornflour/cornstarch together until smooth. Pour over the chicken strips and mix well until coated evenly. Leave to marinate in the refrigerator for at least 20 minutes.

2   When ready to cook, drain the chicken and reserve. Heat a wok or large frying pan, add the oil and, when hot, add the chicken and stir-fry for 1–2 minutes, or until the chicken has turned white. Using a slotted spoon, remove from the wok and reserve.

3   Wipe the wok and return to the heat. Add chicken stock, lemon juice, soy sauce, Chinese rice wine or sherry, sugar, garlic and chilli flakes and bring to the boil. Blend remaining cornflour with 1 tablespoon water and stir into the stock. Simmer for 1 minute.

4   Return the chicken to the wok and continue simmering for a further 2–3 minutes, or until the chicken is tender and the sauce has thickened. Garnish with lemon strips and red chilli slices. Serve immediately.

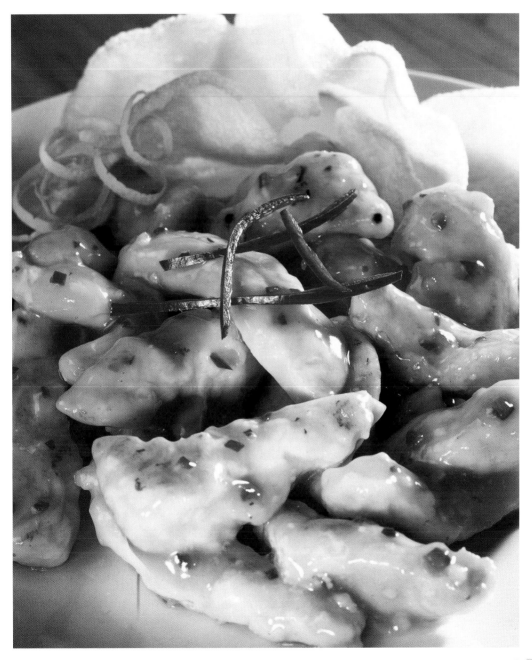

Cakes & Desserts

There are a host of lemon-flavoured desserts, but
even used simply with pancakes, rice-pudding,
cheesecake and ice-cream or sorbet the lemon comes
through with that fantastic palate-cleansing taste,
cutting through any heavy flavours. It's always so
good to finish off a meal with something light and
refreshingly lemony. The lemon works brilliantly with
sugar and that's why the lemon is so effective for
meringues and tarts, not to mention delicious cakes
and icings. How amazing that it can be so delicious
and still good for you!

Lemon Drizzle Cupcakes

Makes 12

150 g/5 oz/²/₃ cup (1¼ sticks) butter, softened
150 g/5 oz/³/₄ cup caster/superfine sugar
3 medium/large eggs, beaten
150 g/5 oz/1¹/₃ cups self-raising flour
¹/₂ tsp baking powder
1 lemon

To decorate:

1 lemon
50 g/2 oz/¹/₄ cup caster/superfine sugar

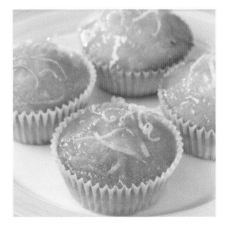

1   Preheat the oven to 180°C/350°F/Gas Mark 4 and line a 12-hole muffin tray/pan with paper cases.

2   Place the butter, sugar and eggs in a bowl and then sift in the flour and baking powder. Finely grate the zest of the lemon into the bowl.

3   Beat together for about 2 minutes, preferably with an electric hand mixer, until pale and fluffy. Spoon into the paper cases and bake for 25 minutes until firm and golden. Cool on a wire rack.

4   To make the topping, cut the zest from the other lemon into thin strips and set aside. Squeeze the juice from the lemon into a small saucepan. Add the sugar and heat gently until every grain of sugar has dissolved. Add the strips of zest and cool slightly. Spoon the syrup and lemon strips over the cupcakes while still warm. Leave to cool. Keep for 4 days in an airtight container.

Ginger & Lemon Cupcakes

Makes 18

8 tbsp golden/light corn syrup
125 g/4 oz/$^1/_2$ cup (1 stick) block margarine
225 g/8 oz/2 cups plain/all-purpose flour
2 tsp ground ginger
75 g/3 oz sultanas/golden raisins
50 g/2 oz/$^1/_3$ cup soft dark brown sugar
200 ml/7 fl oz/$^3/_4$ cup milk
1 tsp baking powder
1 medium/large egg, beaten

To decorate:

125 g/4 oz/1$^1/_4$ cups golden icing/unbleached
    confectioners' sugar
1 tsp lemon juice
glacé/candied ginger pieces

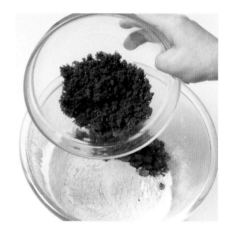

1   Preheat the oven to 180°C/350°F/Gas Mark 4. Line two shallow muffin trays/pans with
    18 paper cases.

2   Place the syrup and margarine in a heavy-based pan and melt together gently. Sift the
    flour and ginger into a bowl, then stir in the sultanas/golden raisins and sugar. Warm the
    milk and stir in the baking powder.

3   Pour the syrup mixture, milk and beaten egg into the dry ingredients and beat until
    smooth. Pour the mixture into a jug.

4   Carefully spoon 2 tablespoons of the mixture into each case (the mixture will be wet). Bake
    for about 30 minutes. Cool in the tins for 10 minutes, then turn out to cool on a wire rack.

5   To decorate, blend the icing/confectioners' sugar with the lemon juice and 1 tablespoon
    warm water to make a thin glacé icing. Drizzle over the top of each cupcake, then top
    with glacé/candied ginger pieces. Leave to set for 30 minutes. Keep in an airtight
    container for up to 5 days.

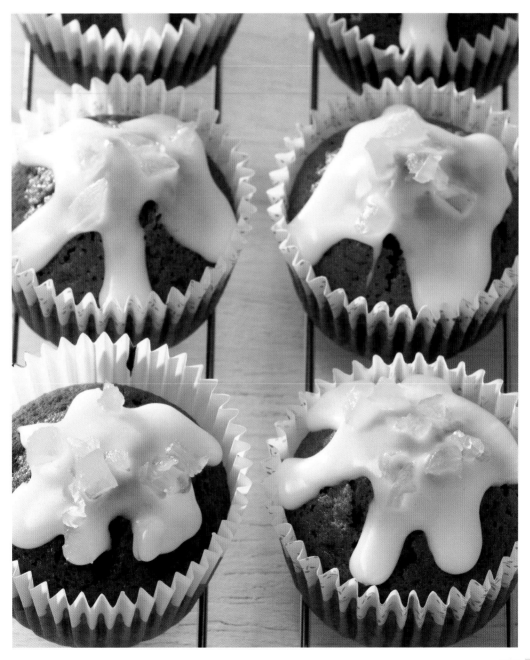

Lemon & Cardamom Cupcakes with Mascarpone Topping

Makes 12

1 tsp cardamom seeds
200 g/7 oz/³/₄ cup plus 2 tbsp (1¹/₄ sticks) butter
50 g/2 oz/¹/₂ cup plain/all-purpose flour
200 g/7 oz/ 2 scant cups self-raising flour
1 tsp baking powder
200 g/7 oz/1 cup caster/superfine sugar
zest of 1 lemon, finely grated
3 medium/large eggs
100 ml/3¹/₂ fl oz/¹/₃ cup natural yogurt
4 tbsp lemon curd

To decorate:

250 g/9 oz tub mascarpone
6 tbsp icing/confectioners' sugar
1 tsp lemon juice
lemon zest strips

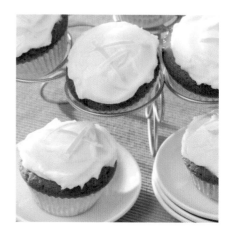

1   Preheat the oven to 180°C/350°F/Gas Mark 4. Line a 12-hole muffin tray/pan with paper cases. Crush the cardamom seeds and remove the outer cases. Melt the butter and leave aside to cool.

2   Sift the flours and baking powder into a bowl and stir in the crushed seeds, sugar and lemon zest. In another bowl, whisk together the eggs and yogurt. Pour into the dry ingredients with the cooled melted butter and beat until combined.

3   Divide half the mixture between the paper cases, put a teaspoon of lemon curd into each, then top with the remaining mixture. Bake for about 25 minutes until golden.

4   To make the topping, beat the mascarpone with the icing/confectioners' sugar and lemon juice. Swirl onto each cupcake and top with lemon strips. Eat fresh on day of baking once decorated or store, undecorated, in an airtight container for up to 2 days and add the topping just before serving.

Lemon Butter Cookies

Makes 14–18

175 g/6 oz/^{3}/$_4$ cup (1^1/$_2$ sticks) butter, softened
75 g/3 oz/^{1}/$_3$ cup caster/superfine sugar
175 g/6 oz/1^1/$_2$ cups plain/all-purpose flour
75 g/3 oz cornflour/cornstarch
zest of 1 lemon, finely grated
2 tbsp caster/superfine sugar, to decorate

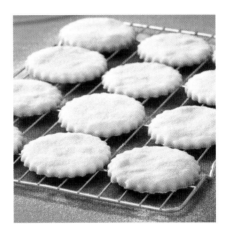

1   Preheat the oven to 170°C/325°F/Gas Mark 3. Grease two baking sheets. Place the butter into a bowl and beat together with the sugar until light and fluffy.

2   Sift in the flour and cornflour/cornstarch, add the lemon zest and mix together with a flat-bladed knife to form a soft dough.

3   Place the dough on a lightly floured surface, knead lightly and roll out thinly. Use biscuit cutters to cut out fancy shapes, re-rolling the trimmings to make more cookies. Carefully lift each cookie onto a baking sheet with a palette knife, then prick lightly with a fork.

4   Bake for 12–15 minutes. Cool on the baking sheets for 5 minutes, then place on a wire rack. Once completely cool, dust with caster/superfine sugar.

Lemon Surprise

Serves 4

6 tbsp low-fat margarine
175 g/6 oz/scant 1 cup caster/superfine sugar
3 small/medium eggs, separated
75 g/3 oz/^{2}/$_3$ cup self-raising flour
450 ml/^{3}/$_4$ pint/1^3/$_4$ cups semi-skimmed/
   low-fat milk
juice of 2 lemons
juice of 1 orange
2 tsp icing/confectioners' sugar
lemon zest, to decorate
sliced strawberries, to serve

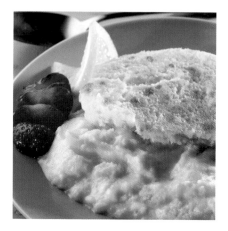

1   Preheat the oven to 190°C/375°F/Gas Mark 5. Lightly oil a deep ovenproof dish.
2   Beat together the margarine and sugar until pale and fluffy. Add the egg yolks, one at a
     time, with 1 tablespoon of the flour and beat well after each addition. Once added, stir
     in the remaining flour. Stir in the milk, 4 tablespoons of the lemon juice and 3
     tablespoons of the orange juice.
3   Whisk the egg whites until stiff and fold into the pudding mixture with a metal spoon or
     rubber spatula until well combined. Pour into the prepared dish.
4   Stand the dish in a roasting tin/pan and pour in just enough boiling water to come
     halfway up the sides of the dish. Bake in the preheated oven for 45 minutes, or until
     well risen and spongy to the touch.
5   Remove the dessert from the oven and sprinkle with the icing/confectioners' sugar.
     Decorate with the lemon zest and serve immediately with the strawberries.

Vanilla & Lemon Panna Cotta with Raspberry Sauce

Serves 6

900 ml/1¹/₂ pints/3³/₄ cups double cream
1 vanilla pod, split
100 g/3¹/₂ oz/¹/₂ cup caster/superfine sugar
zest of 1 lemon
3 sheets gelatine
5 tbsp milk
450 g/1 lb/3 cups raspberries
3–4 tbsp icing/confectioners' sugar, to taste
1 tbsp lemon juice
extra lemon zest, to decorate

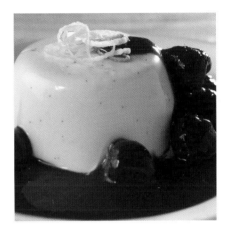

1. Put the cream, vanilla pod and sugar into a saucepan. Bring to the boil, then simmer for 10 minutes until slightly reduced, stirring to prevent scalding. Remove from the heat, stir in the lemon zest and remove the vanilla pod.

2. Soak the gelatine in the milk for 5 minutes, or until softened. Squeeze out any excess milk and add to the hot cream. Stir well until dissolved.

3. Pour the cream mixture into six ramekins or mini pudding moulds and leave in the refrigerator for 4 hours, or until set.

4. Meanwhile, put 175 g/6 oz/1/¹/₂ cups of the raspberries in a food processor with the icing/confectioners' sugar and lemon juice. Blend to a purée then pass the mixture through a sieve. Fold in the remaining raspberries with a metal spoon or rubber spatula and chill in the refrigerator until ready to serve.

5. To serve, dip each of the moulds into hot water for a few seconds, then turn out on to six individual serving plates. Spoon some of the raspberry sauce over and around the panna cotta, decorate with extra lemon zest and serve.

Lemon Meringue Pie

Serves 4–6

175 g/6 oz/1¹/₂ cups plain/all-purpose flour
pinch salt
40 g/1¹/₂ oz lard or white vegetable fat
40 g/1¹/₂ oz/3 tbsp butter or
  block margarine

For the filling:

grated zest and juice of 2 lemons
75 g/3 oz/¹/₃ cup granulated sugar
300 ml/¹/₂ pint/1¹/₄ cups water
40 g/1¹/₂ oz/¹/₃ cup
  cornflour/cornstarch
2 large/extra-large egg yolks

For the topping:

2 large/extra-large egg whites
125 g/4 oz/²/₃ cup caster/superfine sugar

1   Preheat the oven to 200°C/400°F/Gas Mark 6 and place a baking sheet in the oven to heat. Sift the flour and salt into a bowl or a food processor and add the fats, cut into small pieces. Rub in with your fingertips, or process, until the mixture resembles fine crumbs. Mix in 2–3 tablespoons cold water to form a soft dough, then knead lightly until smooth. Grease a 20.5 cm/8 inch round flan tin/tart pan. Roll out the pastry on a lightly floured surface and use to line the dish. Chill for 30 minutes while you make the filling.

2   Put the zest and granulated sugar in a pan with 300 ml/¹/₂ pint/1¹/₄ cups water in a heavy-based pan over a low heat and stir until the sugar has completely dissolved. Blend the cornflour/cornstarch with the lemon juice to a smooth paste, then add to the pan and bring to the boil, stirring all the time. Boil for 2 minutes, then remove from the heat and beat in the egg yolks. Set aside to cool.

3   Prick the pastry case, line with greaseproof paper and pour in baking beans/pie weights. Place on the baking sheet and bake for 10 minutes. Remove from the oven and lift out the paper and beans. Bake the pastry for a further 10 minutes. Remove from the oven, spoon the lemon filling into the pastry case and set aside. Reduce the oven temperature to 150°C/300°F/Gas Mark 2.

4   Whisk the egg whites in a clean, dry bowl until very stiff. Whisk in half the caster/superfine sugar a little at a time, then fold in the remainder. Spread over the lemon filling, making sure it covers the top, right to the edges of the filling. Bake for 30 minutes until the meringue is golden. Leave to 'settle' for 20 minutes before serving, or eat cold on the day of baking.

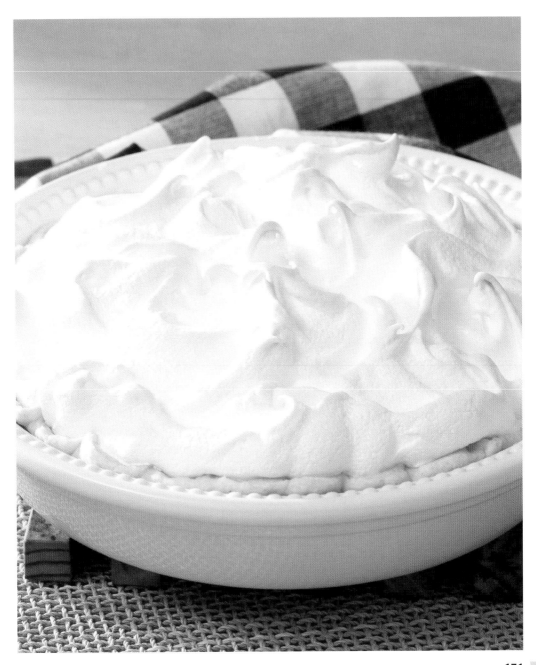

Goats' Cheese & Lemon Tart

Serves 4

For the pastry:

125 g/4 oz/¹/₂ cup (1 stick) butter, cut into small pieces
225 g/8 oz/2 cups plain/all-purpose flour
pinch salt
50 g/2 oz/¹/₄ cup caster/superfine sugar
1 medium/large egg yolk

For the filling:

350 g/12 oz/1¹/₂ cups mild fresh goats' cheese
3 medium/large eggs, beaten
150 g/5 oz/³/₄ cup caster/superfine sugar
grated zest and juice of 3 lemons
450 ml/³/₄ pint/1³/₄ cups double/heavy cream
fresh raspberries, to decorate

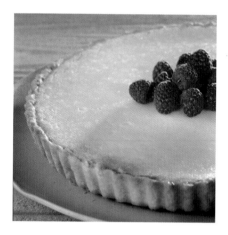

1   Preheat the oven to 200°C/400°F/Gas Mark 6, 15 minutes before baking. Rub the butter
    into the plain/all-purpose flour and salt until the mixture resembles breadcrumbs, then
    stir in the sugar. Beat the egg yolk with 2 tablespoons cold water and add to the
    mixture. Mix together until a dough is formed, then turn the dough out onto a lightly
    floured surface and knead until smooth. Chill in the refrigerator for 30 minutes.

2   Roll the dough out thinly on a lightly floured surface and use to line a 4 cm/1¹/₂ inch
    deep 23 cm/9 inch fluted flan tin/tart pan. Chill in the refrigerator for 10 minutes. Line
    the pastry case/pie crust with greaseproof/wax paper and baking beans/pie weights or
    kitchen foil and bake blind in the preheated oven for 10 minutes. Remove the paper and
    beans or foil. Return to the oven for a further 12–15 minutes until cooked. Leave to
    cool slightly, then reduce the oven temperature to 150°C/300°F/Gas Mark 2.

3   Beat the goats' cheese until smooth. Whisk in the eggs, sugar, lemon zest and juice. Add
    the cream and mix well. Carefully pour the cheese mixture into the pastry case and
    return to the oven. Bake in the oven for 35–40 minutes, or until just set. If it begins to
    brown or swell, open the oven door for 2 minutes. Reduce the temperature to
    120°C/250°F/Gas Mark ¹/₂ and leave the tart to cool in the oven. Chill in the refrigerator
    until cold. Decorate and serve with fresh raspberries.

Chocolate & Lemon Grass Mousse

Serves 4

3 lemon grass stalks, outer leaves removed
200 ml/7 fl oz/³/₄ cup milk
2 sheets gelatine
150 g/5 oz milk chocolate, broken into small pieces
2 medium/large egg yolks
50 g/2 oz/¹/₄ cup caster/superfine sugar
150 ml/¹/₄ pint/²/₃ cup double cream
juice of 2 lemons
1 tbsp caster/superfine sugar
lemon zest, to decorate

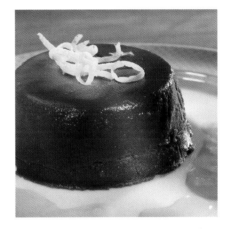

1   Use a wooden spoon to bruise the lemon grass, then cut in half. Pour the milk into a large heavy-based saucepan, add the lemon grass and bring to the boil. Remove from the heat, leave to infuse for 1 hour, then strain. Place the gelatine in a shallow dish, pour over cold water to cover and leave for 15 minutes. Squeeze out excess moisture before use.

2   Place the chocolate in a small bowl set over a saucepan of gently simmering water and leave until melted. Make sure the water does not touch the bowl.

3   Whisk the egg yolks and sugar together until thick, then whisk in the flavoured milk. Pour into a clean saucepan and cook gently, stirring continuously, until the mixture starts to thicken. Remove from the heat, stir in the melted chocolate and gelatine and leave to cool for a few minutes.

4   Whisk the double cream until soft peaks form, then stir into the cooled milk mixture to form a mousse. Spoon into individual ramekins or moulds and leave in the refrigerator for 2 hours or until set.

5   Just before serving, pour the lemon juice into a small saucepan, bring to the boil, then simmer for 3 minutes or until reduced. Add the sugar and heat until dissolved, stirring continuously. Serve the mousse drizzled with the lemon sauce and decorated with lemon zest.

Maple, Pecan & Lemon Loaf

Cuts into 12 slices

350 g/12 oz/2³/₄ cups plain/all-purpose flour
1 tsp baking powder
175 g/6 oz/³/₄ cup (1¹/₂ sticks) butter, cubed
75 g/3 oz/¹/₃ cup caster/superfine sugar
125 g/4 oz/1¹/₄ cups roughly chopped pecan nuts
3 medium/large eggs
1 tbsp milk
finely grated zest of 1 lemon
5 tbsp maple syrup

For the icing:

75 g/3 oz/³/₄ cup icing/confectioners' sugar
1 tbsp lemon juice
25 g/1 oz/¹/₄ cup pecans, roughly chopped

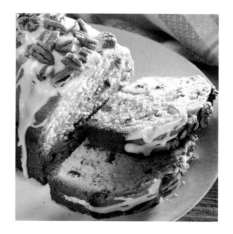

1   Preheat the oven to 170°C/325°F/Gas Mark 3, 10 minutes before baking. Lightly oil and line the base of a 900 g/2 lb loaf tin/pan with nonstick baking parchment.

2   Sift the flour and baking powder into a large bowl. Rub in the butter until the mixture resembles fine breadcrumbs. Stir in the caster/superfine sugar and pecan nuts.

3   Beat the eggs together with the milk and lemon zest. Stir in the maple syrup. Add to the dry ingredients and gently stir in until mixed thoroughly to make a soft dropping consistency.

4   Spoon the mixture into the prepared tin and level the top with the back of a spoon. Bake on the middle shelf of the preheated oven for 50–60 minutes, or until the cake is well risen and lightly browned. If a skewer inserted into the centre comes out clean, then the cake is ready. Leave the cake in the tin for about 10 minutes, then turn out and leave to cool on a wire rack. Carefully remove the lining paper.

5   Sift the icing/confectioners' sugar into a small bowl and stir in the lemon juice to make a smooth icing. Drizzle the icing over the top of the loaf, then scatter with the chopped pecans. Leave to set, slice thickly and serve.

Lemon Bars

Makes 24

175 g/6 oz/1¹/₂ cups plain/all-purpose flour
125 g/4 oz/¹/₂ cup (1 stick) butter
50 g/2 oz/¹/₄ cup caster/superfine sugar
2 tbsp plain/all-purpose flour
¹/₂ tsp baking powder
¹/₄ tsp salt
2 medium/large eggs, lightly beaten
juice and finely grated zest of 1 lemon
sifted icing/confectioners' sugar, to decorate

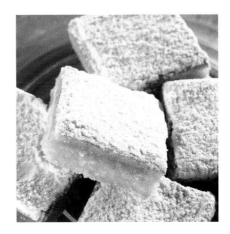

1   Preheat the oven to 170˚C/325˚F/Gas Mark 3, 10 minutes before baking. Lightly oil
    and line a 20.5 cm/8 inch square cake tin/pan with greaseproof/wax paper or baking
    parchment.
2   Rub together the flour and butter until the mixture resembles breadcrumbs. Stir in 4
    tablespoons of the caster/superfine sugar and mix. Turn the mixture into the prepared
    tin and press down firmly. Bake in the preheated oven for 20 minutes until pale golden.
3   Meanwhile, in a food processor, mix together the remaining sugar, the flour, baking
    powder, salt, eggs, lemon juice and zest until smooth. Pour over the prepared base.
4   Transfer to the oven and bake for a further 20–25 minutes until nearly set but still a bit
    wobbly in the centre. Remove from the oven and cool in the tin/pan on a wire rack.
    Dust with icing/confectioners' sugar and cut into squares. Serve cold and store in an
    airtight container.

Baked Lemon & Sultana Cheesecake

Cuts into 10 slices

275 g/9^1/$_2$ oz/1^1/$_3$ cups caster/superfine sugar
50 g/2 oz/4 tbsp butter
50 g/2 oz/^{1}/$_2$ cup self-raising flour
^{1}/$_2$ level tsp baking powder
5 large/extra-large eggs
450 g/1 lb/2 cups cream cheese
40 g/1^1/$_2$ oz/^{1}/$_3$ cup plain/all-purpose flour
grated zest of 1 lemon
3 tbsp fresh lemon juice
150 ml/^{1}/$_4$ pint/^{2}/$_3$ cup crème fraîche/sour cream
75 g/3 oz/^{1}/$_2$ cup sultanas/golden raisins

To decorate:

1 tbsp icing/confectioners' sugar
fresh blackcurrants or blueberries, and mint leaves

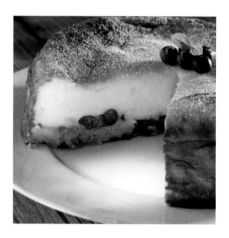

1   Preheat the oven to 170°C/325°F/Gas Mark 3. Oil a 20.5 cm/8 inch loose-bottomed round cake tin/pan with nonstick baking parchment. Beat 50 g/2 oz/^{1}/$_4$ cup of the sugar and the butter together until light and creamy, then stir in the self-raising flour, baking powder and 1 egg. Mix together lightly until well blended. Spoon into the prepared tin and spread the mixture over the base. Separate the 4 remaining eggs and reserve.

2   Blend the cheese in a food processor until soft. Gradually add the yolks and sugar and blend until smooth. Turn into a bowl and stir in the plain/all-purpose flour, zest and juice. Mix lightly before adding the crème fraîche/sour cream and sultanas/golden raisins, stirring well.

3   Whisk the egg whites until stiff, fold into the cheese mixture and pour into the tin. Tap lightly on the work surface to remove any air bubbles. Bake in the preheated oven for about 1 hour, or until golden and firm. Cover lightly if browning too much. Switch the oven off and leave in the oven to cool for 2–3 hours. Remove the cheesecake from the oven. When completely cold, remove from the tin. Sprinkle with icing/confectioners' sugar, decorate with the blackcurrants or blueberries and mint and serve.

Lemon & Apricot Pudding

Serves 4

125 g/4 oz/1 cup dried apricots
3 tbsp orange juice, warmed
50 g/2 oz/4 tbsp butter
125 g/4 oz/$^2/_3$ cup caster/superfine sugar
juice and grated zest of 2 lemons
2 medium/large eggs, separated
100 g/3$^1/_2$ oz/scant 1 cup self-raising flour
300 ml/$^1/_2$ pint/1$^1/_4$ cups milk
custard or fresh cream, to serve

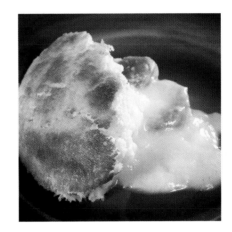

1   Preheat the oven to 180°C/350°F/Gas Mark 4. Oil a 1.2 litre/2 pint/1$^1/_4$ quart pie dish. Soak the apricots in the orange juice for 10–15 minutes, or until most of the juice has been absorbed, then place in the base of the pie dish.

2   Cream the butter and sugar together with the lemon zest until light and fluffy. Beat the egg yolks into the creamed mixture with a spoonful of flour after each addition. Add the remaining flour and beat well until smooth. Stir the milk and lemon juice into the creamed mixture.

3   Whisk the egg whites in a grease-free mixing bowl until stiff and standing in peaks. Fold into the mixture using a metal spoon or rubber spatula. Pour into the prepared dish and place in a baking tray filled with enough cold water to come halfway up the sides of the dish.

4   Bake in the preheated oven for about 45 minutes, or until the sponge is firm and golden brown. Remove from the oven. Serve immediately with the custard or fresh cream.

Chocolate Lemon Tartlets

Makes 10

For the chocolate pastry:

125 g/4 oz /½ cup (1 stick) unsalted butter, softened
65 g/2½ oz/⅓ cup caster/superfine sugar
2 tsp vanilla extract
175 g/6 oz/heaping 1⅓ cups sifted plain/all-purpose flour
40 g/1½ oz/scant ½ cup cocoa powder (unsweetened)

For the filling:

175 ml/6 fl oz/scant ¾ cup double/heavy cream
175 g/6 oz dark/semisweet dark chocolate, chopped
25 g/1 oz/2 tbsp butter, diced
1 tsp vanilla extract
350 g/12 oz/1 cup lemon curd
250 ml/8 fl oz/1 cup prepared custard
250 ml/8 fl oz/1 cup single/light cream
½–1 tsp almond extract

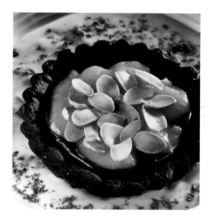

To decorate:

grated chocolate
toasted flaked/slivered almonds

1   To make the pastry dough, put the butter, sugar and vanilla extract into a food processor and blend until creamy. Add the flour and cocoa powder and process until a soft dough forms. Remove the dough, wrap in plastic wrap and chill in the refrigerator for at least an hour.

2   Preheat the oven to 200°C/400°F/Gas Mark 6, 15 minutes before baking. Roll the prepared pastry dough out on a lightly floured surface and use to line ten 7.5 cm/3 inch tartlet tins/pans. Place a small piece of crumpled kitchen foil in each and bake blind in the preheated oven for 12 minutes. Remove from the oven and leave to cool.

3   Bring the cream to the boil, remove from the heat and add the chocolate. Stir until smooth and melted. Beat in the butter and vanilla extract, pour into the tartlets and leave to cool.

4   Beat the lemon curd until soft and spoon a thick layer over the chocolate in each tartlet, spreading gently to the edges. Do not chill in the refrigerator or the chocolate will be too firm.

5   Place the prepared custard into a large bowl and gradually whisk in the cream and almond extract until smooth and runny. To serve, spoon a little custard sauce onto a plate and place a tartlet in the centre. Sprinkle with grated chocolate and almonds, then serve.

Lemon Drizzle Cake

Cuts into 16 squares

125 g/4 oz/¹/₂ cup (1 stick) butter or margarine
175 g/6 oz/1 scant cup caster/superfine sugar
2 large/extra-large eggs
175 g/6 oz/1¹/₂ cups self-raising flour
2 lemons, preferably unwaxed
50 g/2 oz/¹/₄ cup granulated sugar

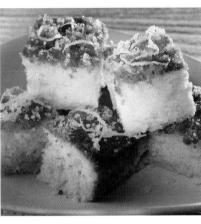

1   Preheat the oven to
    180°C/350°F/Gas Mark 4, 10 minutes
    before baking. Lightly oil and line
    the base of an 18 cm/7 inch square
    cake tin/pan with baking parchment.

2   In a large bowl, cream the butter or
    margarine and caster/superfine sugar together until soft and fluffy.

3   Beat the eggs, then gradually add a little of the egg to the creamed mixture, adding
    1 tablespoon of flour after each addition.

4   Finely grate the zest from one of the lemons and stir into the creamed mixture, beating
    well until smooth. Squeeze the juice from the lemon, strain, then stir into the mixture.
    Spoon into the prepared tin, level the surface and bake in the preheated oven for
    25–30 minutes.

5   Using a zester, remove the zest from the last lemon and mix with 25 g/1 oz of the
    granulated sugar and reserve.

6   Squeeze the juice into a small saucepan. Add the rest of the granulated sugar to the
    lemon juice and heat gently, stirring occasionally. When the sugar has dissolved, simmer
    gently for 3–4 minutes until syrupy.

7   Prick the cake all over with a cocktail stick/toothpick or fine skewer, to allow the syrup to
    soak in. Sprinkle the lemon zest and sugar over the top of the cake, drizzle over the
    syrup and leave to cool in the tin. Cut the cake into squares and serve.

Lemony Coconut Cake

Cuts into 10–12 slices

275 g/10 oz/$2^{1}/_{2}$ cups plain/all-purpose flour

2 tbsp cornflour/cornstarch

1 tbsp baking powder

1 tsp salt

150 g/5 oz/$^{1}/_{2}$ cup white vegetable fat/shortening or soft margarine

275 g/10 oz/$1^{1}/_{3}$ cups caster/superfine sugar

grated zest of 2 lemons

1 tsp vanilla extract

3 large/extra-large eggs

150 ml/$^{1}/_{4}$ pint/$^{2}/_{3}$ cup milk

4 tbsp Malibu or other white rum

450 g/1 lb jar lemon curd

lime zest, to decorate

For the frosting:

275 g/10 oz/$1^{1}/_{3}$ cups caster/superfine sugar

120 ml/4 fl oz/$^{1}/_{2}$ cup water

1 tbsp glucose

$^{1}/_{4}$ tsp salt

1 tsp vanilla extract

3 large/extra-large egg whites

75 g/3 oz/$^{1}/_{2}$ cup desiccated/shredded coconut

1   Preheat the oven to 180°C/350°F/Gas Mark 4, 10 minutes before baking. Lightly oil and flour two 20.5 cm/8 inch nonstick cake tins/pans. Sift the flour, cornflour/cornstarch, baking powder and salt into a large bowl and add the white vegetable fat/shortening or margarine, sugar, lemon zest, vanilla extract, eggs and milk. With an electric whisk on a low speed, beat until blended, adding a little extra milk if the mixture is very stiff. Increase the speed to medium and beat for about 2 minutes. Divide the mixture between the tins and smooth the tops evenly. Bake in the preheated oven for 20–25 minutes, or until the cakes feel firm and are cooked. Remove from the oven and cool before removing from the tins.

2   Put all the ingredients for the frosting, except the coconut, into a heatproof bowl placed over a saucepan of simmering water. (Do not allow the base of the bowl to touch the water.) Using an electric whisk, blend the frosting ingredients on a low speed, then increase the speed to high and beat for 7 minutes until the whites are stiff and glossy. Remove the bowl from the heat and continue beating until cool. Cover with plastic wrap.

3   Using a serrated knife, split the cake layers horizontally in half and sprinkle each cut surface with the rum. Sandwich the cakes together with the lemon curd and press lightly. Spread the top and sides generously with the frosting, swirling and peaking the top. Sprinkle the coconut over the top of the cake and gently press onto the sides to cover. Decorate the cake with the lime zest and serve.

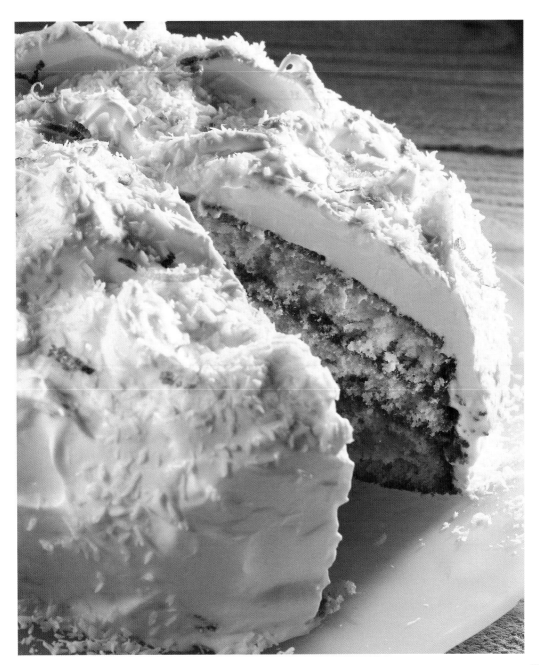

Lemon Fun

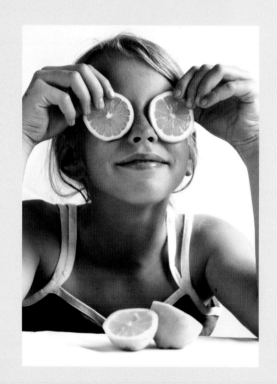

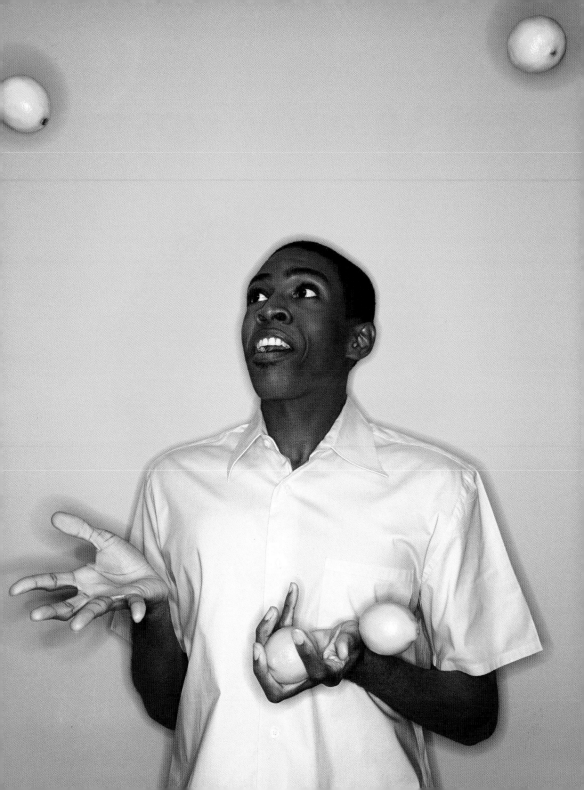

Lemony Tips for Kids

For all its culinary, medicinal and household uses, there is no reason why the lemon can't also be just sheer fun. The lemon is brilliant for a host of exciting science projects, as well as tasty experiments that make full use of the incredible properties of all parts of the lemon. From creating effervescent fizzy powder to making simple lemon batteries, the lemon reveals its versatility and shows its fun side in these exciting projects for kids.

Fun With Lemons

Make Invisible Ink

Use lemon juice to write, but not reveal your secret words. All you need is the juice from a lemon and either a paintbrush or small stick. You could also use a cotton bud as your disposable paintbrush. Dip the paintbrush, cotton bud or stick into the lemon juice and write something on a sheet of paper. You will see nothing. If you now hold the paper up to sunlight or a light bulb, the heat from either of these will cause the hidden words to reveal themselves, as they will slowly turn a pale brown colour. Remember that lemon juice is acidic so it will weaken paper.

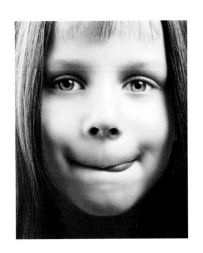

Make Sherbet Lemon

Although this is a wonderful treat and project for the kids, it is also a brilliant adult trip down memory lane – remember sherbet fountains? First you will need to make the sherbet powder, which is simply sugar, bicarbonate of soda (baking soda) and powdered or crystalline citric acid. To test the right proportions you should have two parts sugar to one part citric acid to half a part of bicarbonate of soda.

You could make it extra lemony by putting your mixture in with some lemon peel and leaving it to infuse for a day or two. For maximum effect make sure your sherbet stays dry until you drop it onto your tongue. To prevent the mixture from dissolving and fizzing, dry the lemon peel beforehand to eliminate moisture.

CAUTION: Do not be tempted to squeeze lemon juice onto your mixture as the sherbet will immediately dissolve and fizz if it comes into contact with liquids.

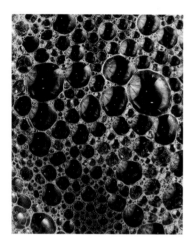

The Lemon Bubbles Project

This is a brilliant science project, but make sure that the kids don't drink this one. Instead they could use it to wash the dishes! Put a teaspoon of bicarbonate of soda (baking soda) into a glass or cup. Add a squirt of washing-up liquid. If you want coloured bubbles, add in one or two drops of food colouring of your choice at this stage. Cut a lemon in half and squeeze out the juice. Then slowly add the lemon juice to your mixture. As the juice hits the mixture bubbles will form and begin to expand out of the glass. You can keep the reaction going by adding some more bicarbonate of soda and lemon juice.

The Lemon Pressure Experiment

For another fun science experiment, cut off the neck of a balloon and the peel of a lemon. Try to cut the lemon peel off as a big slice and shape it to look like perhaps a fish or a boat. Fill a jar with water and place the lemon peel in it. Now stretch the balloon across the top of the jar and seal it with a rubber band. Get the kids to press very gently on the balloon cover. As they press, your lemon shape will sink to the bottom of the water. When they take the pressure off the cover the lemon peel will begin to float to the top of the water.

So what is happening? If you have filled the jar to the very brim then the pressure from the child's hand squashes the tiny air bubbles in the lemon peel to allow water into the peel. This makes it heavier so it sinks. When they take their hand away the air begins to expand once more and the lemon peel floats to the surface.

Make a Battery from a Lemon

Believe it or not, a lemon can also be used as a battery! In fact if you wire up enough lemons together they will even power an LED light.

You will need:
at least one large, fresh, juicy lemon
a galvanized nail (one covered in zinc)
a copper coin

1   Push the galvanized nail into one side of the lemon and the copper coin into the other side of it. Make sure they do not touch each another. You have now created a single-cell battery, with the zinc nail and the copper coin as electrodes. The zinc nail is the negative and the copper coin the positive. The lemon juice acts as an electrolyte. If you were to connect a volt meter to the single-cell lemon battery you will be able to detect a slight voltage.

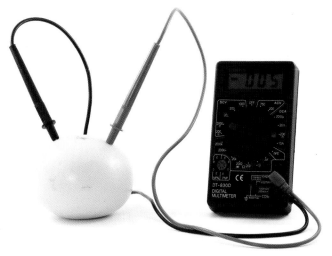

2. You should need around four lemon batteries to be able to power an LED. To light up an LED, use copper wire to connect the positive to the negative from each of your lemon cells. Connect the LED using copper wire. You will need to connect from the zinc nail of the first lemon battery and the copper coin of the last lemon battery. It will glow dimly and is dependent on the quality of the copper, zinc and wire.

Make Your Coins Shine

Dirty old coins can be transformed into bright, shiny copper by simply squeezing out the juice of a lemon and adding a pinch of salt. Leave the coins to soak overnight and in the morning they will look as if they have just been minted.

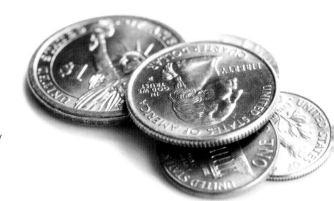

Does a Lemon Float?

To find out the answer, you will need a whole lemon, a bowl of water, a knife and a chopping/cutting board. First get the kids to drop the whole lemon into the water. What happens? The lemon floats! Now get them to take the lemon out of the water and hand it to you. Cut it into quarters and now get them to drop the lemon pieces back into the water. What happens now? The lemon sinks!

Why has this happened? The lemon pulp has absorbed the water and made the lemon wedges heavier, causing them to sink. So the outer skin of the lemon is waterproof. Why would a lemon need to be waterproof? It protects it from harsh weather conditions as it grows and keeps out unwanted, damaging moisture so that the lemon pulp grows succulent and ripe in safety.

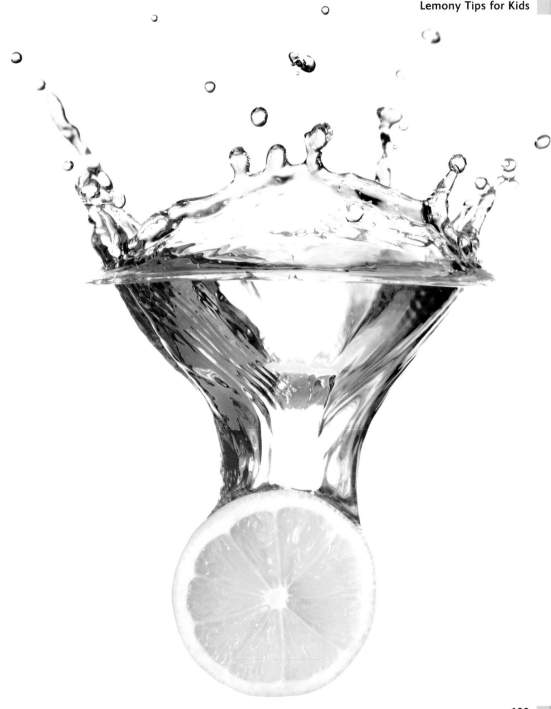

Index

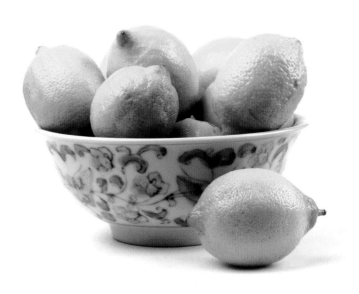